DR. NOWZARADAN DIET PLAN

Beginners-Friendly Transmission of 1200 Calories Approach to a Healthier Life with Expert Strategies, 150-Day Diet Plan and 365-Day Tracking Journal

by

DR. WISPER WALKER

Copyright © 2024 by Dr. Wisper Walker

This book is protected by copyright laws. All rights are reserved. No portion of this book may be reproduced, distributed, or transmitted without the publisher's prior written permission, apart from small extracts in critical reviews and other non-commercial uses authorized by copyright law.

Thank You for Reading!

I hope you will enjoy reading it as much as I enjoyed writing it. Your support means the world to me!

If you find value in these pages, I kindly ask you to consider **leaving an honest review on Amazon.** Your feedback not only helps me improve but also helps other readers discover this book.

TABLE OF CONTENTS

INTRODUCTION — 11

- THE PHILOSOPHY BEHIND — 11
- BENEFITS OF DR. NOWZARADAN'S DIET — 11
- WHAT TO EXPECT — 11
- GETTING STARTED — 11
- DR. NOWZARADAN AND HIS DIET APPROACH — 12

ALL THE SECRETS OF DR. NOWZARADAN'S DIET PLAN — 14

- BIOGRAPHY OF DR. NOWZARADAN — 14
- THE UNDERLYING PHILOSOPHY — 15
- HEALTH BENEFITS AND SCIENTIFIC BACKUP — 17
- SCIENTIFIC EVIDENCE SUPPORTING — 18
- 1200 CALORIES DIET APPROACH — 19
- STRATEGIES FOR EFFECTIVENESS ON THE 1200 CALORIE DIET: ORGANIZING AND SETTING UP MEALS — 20
- SUCCESS STORIES AND TESTIMONIALS — 21
- NUTRITIONAL GUIDELINES FOLLOWING WEIGHT LOSS SURGERY — 24
- TIPS TO ADHERE TO WEIGHT LOSS DIET — 26
- NAVIGATING DINING OUT DURING AN EXTREME WEIGHT LOSS DIET — 28
- DR. NOWZARADAN - LIFE, DIET, AND IMPACT — 30
- WHO DR. NOWZARADAN IS AND WHAT HE IS ABOUT — 31
- WHAT DR. NOWZARADAN'S DIET BROADLY CONSISTS OF — 32
- HOW DR. NOWZARADAN HAS CHANGED THE LIVES OF MANY PEOPLE STRUGGLING WITH OBESITY — 34
- SOME TESTIMONIALS FROM DR. NOWZARADAN'S PATIENTS — 35
- HOW TO START THIS DIET — 36
- THE BASIC BENEFITS IT PROVIDES AND THE SECRETS OF ITS SUCCESS — 37
- THE DISEASES THAT THIS DIET CAN COMBAT — 38
- TRICKS AND TIPS FOR NOT STOPPING FOLLOWING IT — 39
- HOW TO FOLLOW THE DIET EVEN IF YOU HANG OUT WITH FRIENDS AND FAMILY OFTEN — 41

THE MINDSET FOR SUCCESS — 43

- WHY CHANGING MINDSET IS CRITICAL — 44

NEVER LOSE SIGHT OF YOUR GOAL	45
ALREADY SEE YOURSELF AS THE PERSON YOU WANT TO BE	46
ACCEPT CHANGES BECAUSE THEY ARE POSITIVE	47
CHANGE ONE HABIT AT A TIME	47

DR. NOWZARADAN'S DIET PLAN FOR BEGINNERS — 49

BREAKFAST RECIPES	**49**
VEGGIE OMELETTE	49
GREEK YOGURT PARFAIT	50
AVOCADO TOAST	50
PROTEIN PANCAKES	51
BREAKFAST BURRITO	51
OVERNIGHT OATS	52
SMOOTHIE BOWL	52
CHIA SEED PUDDING	53
LUNCH RECIPES	**53**
GRILLED CHICKEN SALAD	53
QUINOA SALAD	54
TURKEY LETTUCE WRAPS	54
VEGGIE STIR-FRY	55
TUNA SALAD	55
LENTIL SOUP	56
QUINOA BOWL	56
STUFFED BELL PEPPERS	57
DINNER RECIPES	**58**
BAKED SALMON	58
TURKEY MEATBALLS	58
STIR-FRIED TOFU	59
CHICKEN STIR-FRY	59
GRILLED VEGGIE SKEWERS	60
SPAGHETTI SQUASH WITH MARINARA	60
CAULIFLOWER FRIED RICE	61
TURKEY CHILI	62
SNACKS	**62**
CELERY STICKS WITH ALMOND BUTTER	62
ALMONDS	63
GREEK YOGURT	63
BABY CARROTS AND HUMMUS	64
APPLE SLICES WITH PEANUT BUTTER	64
COTTAGE CHEESE WITH PINEAPPLE	65

HARD-BOILED EGGS	65
EDAMAME	66
SIDE DISHES	**66**
VEGETABLE SOUP	66
QUINOA PILAF	67
STEAMED BROCCOLI	67
ROASTED BRUSSELS SPROUTS	68
CAULIFLOWER MASH	69
MEAL PLAN CHARTS FOR 30 DAYS	**69**

DR. NOWZARADAN'S MEAL PLAN ON A BUDGET — 72

INTRODUCTION	**72**
BREAKFAST RECIPES	**73**
OATMEAL WITH BANANA SLICES	73
EGG MUFFINS	73
YOGURT WITH GRANOLA	74
BREAKFAST QUESADILLA	74
AVOCADO TOAST WITH HARD-BOILED EGG	75
LUNCH RECIPES	**75**
BLACK BEAN QUESADILLAS	75
QUINOA SALAD WITH VEGGIES	76
RICE AND BEAN BOWL	77
PASTA PRIMAVERA	77
DINNER RECIPES	**78**
SPAGHETTI AGLIO E OLIO	78
BAKED CHICKEN DRUMSTICKS	79
ONE-POT CHILI	79
STUFFED BELL PEPPERS WITH RICE AND BEANS	80
BAKED FISH FILLETS	81
VEGETABLE PASTA BAKE	81
BEAN AND VEGETABLE CASSEROLE	82
SNACKS	**83**
POPCORN: AIR-POPPED POPCORN WITH HERBS OR NUTRITIONAL YEAST	83
CARROT STICKS WITH HUMMUS	83
RICE CAKES WITH ALMOND BUTTER	84
TRAIL MIX	84
SIDE DISHES	**85**
ROASTED VEGETABLES	85
BLACK BEAN SALAD	85
MASHED SWEET POTATOES	86

CUCUMBER TOMATO SALAD	86
MEAL PLAN CHARTS FOR 30 DAYS	**86**

DR. NOWZARADAN'S LOW CARB HIGH PROTEIN RECIPES — 90

INTRODUCTION	**90**
BREAKFAST RECIPES	**90**
SPINACH AND FETA OMELETTE	90
CRUSTLESS QUICHE WITH BACON AND CHEDDAR	91
GREEK YOGURT PARFAIT WITH BERRIES AND ALMONDS	91
VEGGIE BREAKFAST CASSEROLE	92
LOW-CARB PROTEIN PANCAKES	92
SMOKED SALMON AND AVOCADO TOAST	93
COTTAGE CHEESE AND BERRY BOWL	93
EGG AND VEGGIE MUFFIN CUPS	94
LUNCH RECIPES	**94**
GRILLED CHICKEN CAESAR SALAD	94
TURKEY AND AVOCADO WRAP	95
TUNA SALAD LETTUCE WRAPS	95
ZUCCHINI NOODLE STIR-FRY WITH CHICKEN	96
EGG SALAD STUFFED BELL PEPPERS	96
SHRIMP AND VEGGIE SKEWERS	97
CAULIFLOWER FRIED RICE WITH TOFU	97
GREEK CHICKEN SALAD BOWL	98
DINNER RECIPES	**98**
BAKED SALMON WITH ASPARAGUS	98
TURKEY MEATBALLS WITH ZOODLES	99
SPAGHETTI SQUASH WITH CHICKEN ALFREDO	99
BEEF AND BROCCOLI STIR-FRY	100
STUFFED PORTOBELLO MUSHROOMS	100
GRILLED LEMON HERB CHICKEN	101
CAULIFLOWER CRUST PIZZA	102
BAKED COD WITH TOMATO BASIL RELISH	102
SNACKS	**103**
GREEK YOGURT AND BERRY SMOOTHIE	103
PROTEIN-PACKED DEVILED EGGS	103
COTTAGE CHEESE AND TOMATO SLICES	104
TURKEY AND CHEESE ROLL-UPS	104
ROASTED CHICKPEAS	104
CHEESE AND VEGGIE PLATTER	105
PROTEIN ENERGY BALLS	105

SIDE DISHES — 106
- Chicken and Vegetable Soup — 106
- Broccoli Cheddar Soup — 106
- Caprese Salad — 107
- Roasted Brussels Sprouts with Bacon — 107
- Eggplant Parmesan — 108
- Cucumber Avocado Salad — 108
- **Meal Plan Charts for 30 Days** — 109

LOW-CALORIE KETO RECIPES — 112

- Introduction to the Ketogenic Diet — 112
- Health Benefits of the Ketogenic Diet — 113
- Benefits of the Keto Diet — 113
- **Keto Breakfast Recipes** — 115
- Spinach and Mushroom Crustless Quiche — 115
- Keto Avocado Egg Cups — 116
- Zucchini Fritters with Sour Cream — 116
- Egg and Bacon Muffin Cups — 117
- Keto Green Smoothie — 117
- Almond Flour Pancakes with Berries — 118
- **Keto Lunch Recipes** — 119
- Keto Chicken Salad Lettuce Wraps — 119
- Keto Turkey Club Lettuce Wraps — 119
- Keto Taco Salad — 120
- Keto Egg Roll in a Bowl — 120
- Keto Cauliflower Fried Rice — 121
- Keto Avocado Tuna Salad — 122
- Keto Turkey and Cheese Roll-Ups — 122
- Keto Greek Salad with Grilled Chicken — 123
- **Keto Dinner Recipes** — 123
- Keto Baked Salmon with Lemon Butter Sauce — 123
- Keto Cauliflower Crust Pizza — 124
- Keto Garlic Butter Shrimp Scampi — 125
- Keto Chicken Alfredo Zoodles — 125
- Keto Stuffed Bell Peppers — 126
- Keto Beef and Broccoli Stir-Fry — 127
- Keto Spaghetti Squash with Meatballs — 127
- **Keto Snack Recipes** — 128
- Keto Cheese Crisps — 128
- Keto Guacamole with Veggie Sticks — 129

KETO FAT BOMBS	129
KETO STUFFED MINI BELL PEPPERS	130
KETO ZUCCHINI CHIPS	130
KETO BUFFALO CHICKEN DIP	131
KETO PECAN PIE BARS	131
KETO SOUP RECIPES	**132**
KETO CHICKEN ZOODLE SOUP	132
KETO CREAM OF BROCCOLI SOUP	133
KETO BEEF AND CABBAGE SOUP	133
KETO CAULIFLOWER CHEESE SOUP	134
KETO CHICKEN AND MUSHROOM SOUP	134
KETO ITALIAN SAUSAGE SOUP	135
KETO CREAMY ASPARAGUS SOUP	136
KETO SEAFOOD CHOWDER	136
MEAL PLAN CHARTS FOR 30 DAYS	**137**

RECIPES SUITABLE FOR DR. NOWZARADAN'S DIET — 140

BREAKFAST RECIPES:	**140**
VEGGIE EGG WHITE SCRAMBLE	140
BERRY SMOOTHIE BOWL	140
SPINACH AND TOMATO FRITTATA	141
GREEK YOGURT WITH NUTS AND SEEDS	141
OVERNIGHT CHIA PUDDING	142
BAKED APPLE OATMEAL	142
MUSHROOM AND KALE BREAKFAST SKILLET	143
LUNCH RECIPES	**143**
GRILLED CHICKEN AND VEGGIE WRAP	143
QUINOA AND BLACK BEAN SALAD	144
CHICKPEA AND CUCUMBER SALAD	144
ASIAN CHICKEN LETTUCE WRAPS	145
SHRIMP AND AVOCADO SALAD	145
SPICY LENTIL SOUP	146
DINNER RECIPES	**147**
BAKED COD WITH ROASTED VEGETABLES	147
TURKEY AND ZUCCHINI MEATBALLS	147
STUFFED EGGPLANT BOATS	148
GARLIC LEMON CHICKEN WITH ASPARAGUS	149
SALMON AND SPINACH SALAD	149
BEEF AND VEGETABLE STIR-FRY	150
CAULIFLOWER RICE WITH GRILLED SHRIMP	150

CHICKEN AND VEGGIE SKEWERS	151
SNACK RECIPES	**152**
MIXED NUTS	152
TUNA SALAD CUCUMBER BITES	152
SOUP RECIPES	**153**
VEGETABLE SOUP	153
CHICKEN AND VEGETABLE SOUP	153
TOMATO BASIL SOUP	154
MINESTRONE SOUP	154
SPLIT PEA SOUP	155
MUSHROOM BARLEY SOUP	155
MEAL PLAN CHARTS FOR 30 DAYS	**156**

365-DAY TRACKING JOURNAL FOR WEIGHT LOSS — 159

DAILY TRACKING	**160**
WEEKLY REFLECTION	**161**
MONTHLY REVIEW	**162**
365-DAY REFLECTION	**163**
HOW TO USE THE 52-WEEK JOURNAL AND THE IMPORTANCE OF TRACKING PROGRESS	**165**
IMPORTANCE OF TRACKING PROGRESS	165
HOW TO USE THE JOURNAL	165

INTRODUCTION

WELCOME TO YOUR HEALTH TRANSFORMATION JOURNEY

Setting out to enhance your well-being and health is a brave and admirable choice. With the help of Dr. Nowzaradan's diet, you can lose a lot of weight and improve your general health. Recognized for his contributions to the television program "My 600-lb Life," Dr. Nowzaradan has created a tried-and-true weight-loss strategy that prioritizes moderation, a healthy diet, and regular observation.

THE PHILOSOPHY BEHIND

Dr. Nowzaradan's Diet is based on the principle that sustainable weight loss can be achieved through a balanced, calorie-controlled diet that provides all the essential nutrients your body needs. This diet focuses on:

Reducing Calorie Intake: The diet restricts daily calorie consumption to 1200 calories or fewer based on medical recommendations and specific needs.
High Protein, Low Carb: Stressing high-protein diets aids fat loss and muscle maintenance. Consuming fewer carbohydrates makes reducing total calorie intake and controlling blood sugar levels easier.
Balanced Nutrition: Ensuring that your intake of vitamins, minerals, and other nutrients is balanced to maintain your general health.
Portion Control: Learning to manage portion sizes to avoid overeating and to create sustainable eating habits.

BENEFITS OF DR. NOWZARADAN'S DIET

Effective Weight Loss: The regimented diet promotes healthy, steady weight loss.
Improved Health: This diet can improve blood pressure, cholesterol, blood sugar control, and other health markers by emphasizing foods high in nutrients.
Enhanced Energy Levels: Eating a balanced diet rich in nutrients can make you feel more alive and energetic.
Improved Relationship with Food: Mindful eating and portion management techniques can help cultivate a better relationship with food, which lowers the risk of binge eating.

WHAT TO EXPECT

Following Dr. Nowzaradan's Diet requires commitment and dedication, but the rewards are worth it. You can expect:

Structured Meal Plans: Structured meal plans organize and guide meals for breakfast, lunch, supper, snacks, and even side dishes and soups.
Diverse Recipes: A selection of mouthwatering dishes that satisfy a range of palates and dietary requirements, guaranteeing that you enjoy your meals while consuming a sensible amount of calories.
Support and Guidance: Useful advice, inspirational ideas, and resources to keep you on course, including a 52-week notebook to monitor your development.

GETTING STARTED

To begin your journey with Dr. Nowzaradan's Diet:

Set Clear Goals: Identify your desired outcomes, such as a particular weight reduction goal, enhanced health indicators, or improved eating practices.
Plan Your Meals: Stay within your calorie limitations by prepping your meals ahead of time using the meal plans and recipes provided.
Track Your Progress: Use the 52-week diary to track your daily food intake, physical activity, water intake, sleep patterns, and emotional state. Continually assess your progress and make necessary adjustments to your plan.
Stay Committed: Reliability is essential. Remain committed to your objectives, ask for help when needed, and acknowledge and appreciate your progress.

DR. NOWZARADAN AND HIS DIET APPROACH

BIOGRAPHY OF DR. NOWZARADAN

Renowned Iranian-American surgeon Dr. Younan Nowzaradan, also referred to as Dr. Now, specializes in bariatric and vascular surgery. Dr. Nowzaradan was born in Tehran, Iran, in 1944, and he immigrated to the US to continue his medical profession in 1970 after earning his medical degree from the University of Tehran. He finished his medical education in the US, where he refined his abilities and found a passion for treating patients with extreme obesity. Due to his participation in the TLC reality television series "My 600-lb Life," where he assisted several patients in losing a considerable amount of weight and improving their quality of life, Dr. Nowzaradan became well-known.

THE UNDERLYING PHILOSOPHY OF DR. NOWZARADAN'S DIET

Dr. Nowzaradan's diet philosophy is based on the idea that behavioral modifications combined with a strict low-calorie diet can result in significant weight loss. He highlights the importance of limiting calorie consumption and consuming foods high in nutrients to aid in weight loss. Dr. Nowzaradan suggests eating a well-balanced diet high in protein and low in fats and carbohydrates to maintain lean muscle mass while losing weight and encouraging satiety. His method guarantees long-term weight management success while preparing patients for bariatric surgery.

HEALTH BENEFITS AND SCIENTIFIC BACKUP OF DR. NOWZARADAN'S DIET

Dr. Nowzaradan's diet has significant health benefits, especially for those with morbid obesity and associated comorbidities. Scientific research has shown that low-calorie, high-protein diets are effective in promoting weight loss, lowering the risk of chronic illnesses like type 2 diabetes, hypertension, and cardiovascular disease, and enhancing metabolic health in general. Following Dr. Nowzaradan's dietary recommendations can help patients lose significant weight, improving their quality of life, mobility, and pain management.

DR. NOWZARADAN'S 1200 CALORIES DIET APPROACH

The 1200-calorie daily consumption recommendation is the cornerstone of Dr. Nowzaradan's diet plan. This low-calorie diet aims to induce a significant calorie deficit, forcing the body to burn fat reserves for energy. Lean protein sources, including chicken, fish, lentils, and a range of non-starchy vegetables, are prioritized in the diet. It restricts the intake of harmful fats and carbs, mainly processed sweets and wheat. Patients can attain quick weight loss, qualifying them for bariatric surgery and laying the groundwork for long-term weight control by adhering to a rigorous diet of 1200 calories.

SUCCESS STORIES AND TESTIMONIALS OF DR. NOWZARADAN'S DIET

Numerous patients have shared their transformational experiences due to Dr. Nowzaradan's nutrition approach, leading to severalseveral success stories. Patient testimonials highlight substantial weight loss and enhancements to general happiness, mental and physical health, and physical wellness. These anecdotes demonstrate the efficacy of Dr. Nowzaradan's approach and provide a potent inspiration for those starting weight reduction journeys.

NUTRITIONAL GUIDELINES FOLLOWING WEIGHT LOSS SURGERY

Dr. Nowzaradan gives patients special dietary instructions after surgery to guarantee ongoing weight loss and avoid problems. These recommendations stress the value of modest, frequent meals that are low in fat and sugar and high in protein. Patients are encouraged to drink lots of water and abstain from alcohol and carbonated drinks since proper hydration is essential. Patients who follow these recommendations can better sustain their weight loss and make lifestyle changes for the better.

TIPS TO ADHERE TO WEIGHT LOSS DIET

Adhering to a rigid eating plan for weight loss can be difficult. Meal planning, mindful eating, and goal-setting are just a few helpful advice Dr. Nowzaradan provides to patients to help them stay on course. He advises patients to establish a support network with friends, family, and support organizations to keep them accountable and motivated. They are developing appropriate coping strategies and overcoming obstacles in the program.

NAVIGATING DINING OUT DURING AN EXTREME WEIGHT LOSS

and supporting organizations to keep accountable and motivated is challenging for people following a tight diet. When dining out, Dr. Nowzaradan counsels his patients to choose dishes that meet their dietary requirements. This entails avoiding high-calorie appetizers and desserts, asking for dressings and sauces on the side, and selecting protein sources that are grilled or steamed. Patients can enjoy dining out without jeopardizing their efforts to lose weight by being organized and making thoughtful decisions.

DR. NOWZARADAN - LIFE, DIET, AND IMPACT

The influence of Dr. Nowzaradan goes beyond his clinical work. He has come to represent change and hope for those who are battling extreme obesity. His firm yet sympathetic approach has motivated Numerous individuals to take charge of their health and reach their weight loss objectives. Through his publications, television programs, and public appearances, Dr. Nowzaradan is inspiring people to lead healthier lives.

Dr. Nowzaradan's comprehensive diet plan, which helps people lose weight, is based on a low-calorie, high-protein diet and behavioral changes. His approaches have produced many success stories and are supported by empirical data. Those who adhere to his rules and advice can overcome the difficulties of losing weight and start a life-changing path toward improved health and well-being.

ALL THE SECRETS OF DR. NOWZARADAN'S DIET PLAN

The success of Dr. Nowzaradan's eating plan can be attributed to several fundamental ideas. Among them are:

Caloric Restriction: Limit daily consumption to approximately 1200 calories to produce a sizable deficit.
High Protein Intake: Giving lean protein sources priority to maintain muscle mass and encourage satiety.
Low Carbohydrate and Fat: Cutting back on sugar and bad fats to avoid consuming too many calories.
Balanced Nutrition: Ensure the diet has the minerals and vitamins to promote general health.
Behavioral Changes: Patients should be encouraged to take up healthy diet and lifestyle practices for long-term success.

BIOGRAPHY OF DR. NOWZARADAN

A well-respected and well-known figure in the medical community, especially in vascular and bariatric surgery, is Dr. Younan Nowzaradan, also lovingly referred to as Dr. Now. During his long career, he has committed himself to assisting the highly obese in losing weight and getting healthier.

EARLY LIFE AND EDUCATION

Iran's Tehran was where Dr. Nowzaradan was born on October 11, 1944. From a young age, he had a strong interest in medicine, which inspired him to enroll in the esteemed University of Tehran to seek a medical degree. In 1970, he earned a Doctor of Medicine (MD) degree, showcasing remarkable academic ability and a solid dedication to his chosen vocation.

MOVE TO THE UNITED STATES AND MEDICAL TRAINING

Dr. Nowzaradan relocated to the US for possibilities and more sophisticated medical training. After finishing his surgical internship at St. Johns Hospital in Detroit, Michigan, he went to St. Thomas Hospital in Nashville, Tennessee, for his surgical residency. Additionally, Dr. Nowzaradan finished his residency in cardiovascular surgery at Houston, Texas's Texas Heart Institute. He received thorough training in patient care and surgical methods from these encounters.

CAREER AND SPECIALIZATION

Throughout his multi-decade career, Dr. Nowzaradan has made significant advances in bariatric and vascular surgery. He specializes in weight loss surgery for morbidly obese people and holds a board certification in general surgery. He is skilled in carrying out complex surgeries such as laparoscopic surgery, sleeve gastrectomy, and gastric bypass.

CONTRIBUTIONS TO BARIATRIC SURGERY

Dr. Nowzaradan's most well-known contribution is his groundbreaking work in bariatric surgery, which aims to assist patients with extreme obesity achieve long-term weight loss. His method addresses the psychological as well as the physical components of obesity by combining surgical surgery, a rigorous diet, and continued support. Numerous patients' lives have been entirely changed by Dr. Nowzaradan's treatments, which have helped them drop a large amount of weight and enhance their general health and quality of life.

"MY 600-LB LIFE"

Due to his participation in the TLC reality television series "My 600-lb Life," which debuted in 2012, Dr. Nowzaradan became well-known worldwide. The program chronicles the experiences of patients who weigh more than 600 pounds as they work with Dr. Nowzaradan to reduce their weight through lifestyle modifications and surgery. Viewers have responded well to his honest but caring style, making him a well-liked character in the reality TV world. The program has raised awareness of the difficulties experienced by those who are highly obese, as well as the life-changing potential of bariatric surgery.

PUBLICATIONS AND RESEARCH

Besides his clinical practice, Dr. Nowzaradan has contributed writing and research to the medical community. He authorizes multiple papers and articles about obesity, weight loss, and minimally invasive surgery. His work has improved patient outcomes from surgery and advanced our understanding of the advantages of bariatric surgery.

PERSONAL PHILOSOPHY AND LEGACY

The core of Dr. Nowzaradan's concept is the conviction that each patient deserves compassionate care and the chance to have a better life. He highlights the significance of treating obesity through a multidisciplinary strategy that includes long-term follow-up, dietary modifications, psychological support, and surgery. He has gained great respect and appreciation for his steadfast commitment to his patient's well-being and dedication to them.

Dr. Nowzaradan's influence goes beyond his clinical work. He is now a spokesperson for obesity awareness and encourages those dealing with weight problems. His studies show that substantial and long-lasting weight loss is achievable with the correct assistance and perseverance.

THE UNDERLYING PHILOSOPHY

The diet philosophy of Dr. Younan Nowzaradan is a comprehensive method designed to help people who are very obese lose a large amount of weight while also enhancing their long-term health and well-being. His approach is grounded on medical science and real-world experience, combining stringent dietary recommendations with behavioral modifications. The following are the central tenets of Dr. Nowzaradan's diet:

CALORIC RESTRICTION

Calorie restriction is a cornerstone of Dr. Nowzaradan's diet plan. Typically, the diet caps daily calorie intake at approximately 1200. This restriction is essential to generate a sizable calorie deficit and push the body to burn stored fat for energy. Patients can lose weight quickly by ingesting fewer calories than their bodies require, which is crucial for getting ready for bariatric surgery.

HIGH PROTEIN INTAKE
Dr. Nowzaradan stresses the value of eating a diet rich in protein. Protein is essential for inducing satiety, which helps patients feel fuller for extended periods and consume fewer calories overall. Protein is also necessary to maintain lean muscle mass while losing weight. Because lean muscle burns more calories at rest than fat tissue, it is metabolically active and can help to maintain a higher metabolic rate.

LOW CARBOHYDRATES AND FATS
The diet drastically decreases consumption of lipids and carbohydrates, mainly processed sweets and bad fats. Carbohydrates, incredibly refined carbohydrates found in white bread and sugary snacks, can cause blood sugar to rise and stimulate insulin secretion, encouraging fat storage. By limiting the amount of carbohydrates consumed, the diet helps to lower cravings and normalize blood sugar levels. When consumed in moderation, healthy fats promote general health without adding to an excessive caloric intake.

BALANCED NUTRITION
The diet guarantees that patients receive adequate nutrition even with calorie restriction by including a range of nutrient-dense foods. Non-starchy veggies, lean proteins, small amounts of whole grains, and healthy fats provide essential vitamins and minerals. This well-rounded strategy promotes general health and helps avoid dietary deficits.

BEHAVIORAL CHANGES
In addition to what patients eat, Dr. Nowzaradan's diet considers their eating habits and relationship with food. He stresses the significance of forming wholesome food habits and adopting long-term lifestyle adjustments. This involves mindful eating techniques, including eating deliberately, observing signs of hunger and fullness, and refraining from emotional eating. Patients are urged to recognize and treat the psychological causes of their overindulgence in food.

PREPARATION FOR SURGERY AND LONG-TERM SUCCESS
Dr. Nowzaradan's diet helps many patients prepare for bariatric surgery. By decreasing weight before the procedure, patients can lower their risk of surgery and achieve better results—more minor liver results from diet, which makes the surgery safer and more accessible—additionally, starting the diet before surgery aids in developing self-control and routines required for long-term success following surgery.

SUPPORT AND ACCOUNTABILITY
Dr. Nowzaradan is aware that reaching weight loss objectives requires accountability and support. He advises patients to create a support network via friends, family, or support organizations. The nutrition plan must also include frequent check-ins and follow-up appointments, giving patients the direction and encouragement to stick to it.

EDUCATION AND EMPOWERMENT
A fundamental element of Dr. Nowzaradan's diet philosophy is education. Patients receive education regarding dietary effects on their bodies, portion sizes, and nutrition. If they comprehend the dietary tenets, patients may take charge of their health and make educated decisions.

LONG-TERM HEALTH AND WELL-BEING

Dr. Nowzaradan's diet supports long-term health and well-being rather than short-term weight loss. By changing their diet and lifestyle, patients can lower their chance of developing chronic illnesses like type 2 diabetes, hypertension, and cardiovascular disease. Reduction of pain, increased mobility, and improved quality of life are other essential advantages of effective weight loss.

Dr. Nowzaradan's diet philosophy is a comprehensive weight loss and health improvement approach incorporating behavioral modifications, stringent dietary requirements, and continuous support. He presents a complete diet plan that addresses extreme obesity by emphasizing high protein consumption, balanced nutrition, sustainable lifestyle adjustments, and caloric restriction.

HEALTH BENEFITS AND SCIENTIFIC BACKUP

Research has shown that Dr. Nowzaradan's diet, which is mainly for people who are highly obese, has some positive health effects. This diet helps people lose weight and enhances their physical and emotional well-being. It strongly emphasizes calorie restriction, high protein intake, and balanced nutrition. The primary health advantages of Dr. Nowzaradan's diet, together with the supporting scientific data, are as follows:

SIGNIFICANT WEIGHT LOSS

Significant weight loss is the main objective of Dr. Nowzaradan's diet, which is essential for people getting ready for bariatric surgery. By causing a calorie deficit through calorie restriction, the body is compelled to burn fat reserves for energy. Several studies have demonstrated that low-calorie diets help people lose weight quickly. A study in "The American Journal of Clinical Nutrition" discovered that following a low-calorie diet for three to six months can result in an average weight loss of 15 to 25 percent of one's starting body weight.

BETTER HEALTH OF THE METABOLIC PROCESS

Dr. Nowzaradan's diet lowers insulin resistance and stabilizes blood sugar, contributing to better metabolic health. Low-carbohydrate and high-protein diets help stabilize blood glucose levels, reducing the risk of type 2 diabetes. Studies in "Diabetes Care" show that low-calorie diets can significantly enhance glycemic control and insulin sensitivity in obese people.

REDUCTION IN CARDIOVASCULAR RISK FACTORS

One of the main risk factors for cardiovascular conditions, such as atherosclerosis, dyslipidemia, and hypertension, is obesity. Dr. Nowzaradan's diet encourages weight loss and improves lipid profiles, which help reduce these risks. Research has indicated that diets high in protein and low in calories can lower blood pressure, triglycerides, and LDL cholesterol while raising HDL cholesterol. Research published in the "Journal of the American College of Cardiology" showed that dietary interventions leading to significant weight loss can lower cardiovascular risk factors by 20–30%.

ENHANCED MOBILITY AND REDUCED PAIN
Dr. Nowzaradan's diet can help patients lose weight, which can significantly improve mobility and lessen discomfort from obesity-related illnesses like osteoarthritis. Carrying too much weight puts extra strain on joints, especially the hips and knees, which can cause pain and limited movement. Studies published in "Arthritis Care & Research" demonstrate that people with knee osteoarthritis can have notable improvements in pain and function with even modest weight loss.

IMPROVED RESPIRATORY FUNCTION AND SLEEP APNEA
Obstructive sleep apnea (OSA) and other respiratory problems are frequently associated with obesity. Losing weight can improve respiratory mechanics and lessen the severity of OSA by lowering fat deposits in the upper airway. According to a study published in the "American Journal of Respiratory and Critical Care Medicine," losing weight can significantly lessen the severity of sleep apnea symptoms.

PSYCHOLOGICAL BENEFITS
Dr. Nowzaradan's diet has the potential to improve mental health in addition to physical health. Low self-esteem, anxiety, and sadness are frequently linked to obesity. Control overweight can enhance one's sense of self-worth, body image, and general psychological health. A study that was published in "Obesity Reviews" emphasized the benefits of weight loss on mental health and found that obese people who lost weight had significantly fewer symptoms of anxiety and depression.

LONG-TERM HEALTH BENEFITS
Dr. Nowzaradan's diet can help people lose and maintain weight over time, which can have long-term health benefits, such as a lowered chance of developing chronic illnesses like type 2 diabetes, heart disease, stroke, and some malignancies. A thorough analysis published in The Lancet discovered that long-term weight loss is linked to a lower chance of chronic illness development and a longer life expectancy.

SCIENTIFIC EVIDENCE SUPPORTING

Dr. Nowzaradan's diet is supported scientifically by well-established concepts in nutrition and metabolic health:

CALORIC RESTRICTION:
Much research demonstrates that calorie restriction helps encourage weight loss and enhance metabolic health. Low-calorie diets lower blood pressure, improve insulin sensitivity, and reduce fat mass.

HIGH PROTEIN INTAKE:
Research has shown that diets high in protein increase metabolic rate, maintain lean muscle mass during weight loss, and encourage satiety. Consuming protein also contributes to maintaining muscle mass, essential for long-term weight control.

LOW CARBOHYDRATE CONSUMPTION:
Cutting back on carbohydrates, mainly processed sweets, helps regulate blood sugar levels and lessens insulin surges, which can lead to fat storage. Low-carb diets have been linked to higher early weight reduction than low-fat diets.

BALANCED NUTRITION:
A diet of vital nutrients keeps deficits at bay and promotes general health. Non-starchy veggies, lean meats, and healthy fats contain the vitamins, minerals, and fiber required for suitable biological activities.

A wealth of scientific evidence substantiates the efficacy of Dr. Nowzaradan's diet in producing notable weight reduction and enhancing a range of health metrics. The diet provides a comprehensive strategy to address obesity and related health issues because of its emphasis on calorie restriction, high protein intake, and balanced nutrition. According to Dr. Nowzaradan's recommendations, people's physical and mental health can significantly improve, and their quality of life can be enhanced.

1200 CALORIES DIET APPROACH

Essential Elements in the 1200 Calorie Diet

CALORIC RESTRICTION
By capping daily calorie intake at 1200, the diet produces a significant calorie deficit that compels the body to use fat reserves for energy. This amount of calories is adequate to support noticeable weight loss while supplying essential nutrients.

HIGH PROTEIN INTAKE
Protein is an essential component of the diet since it increases satiety and helps to maintain muscle mass while losing weight. Lean meats (turkey, chicken), fish, eggs, low-fat dairy products, and legumes are familiar protein sources.

LOW CARBOHYDRATES
Minimize your carbohydrate intake to prevent insulin and blood sugar surges, which might cause you to store fat. The diet focuses on low-glycemic index carbs, such as non-starchy vegetables and small amounts of whole grains.

LIMITED FATS
It is recommended that people consume moderate amounts of healthy fats, mostly from nuts, avocados, and olive oil. Limiting trans and saturated fats lowers the risk of cardiovascular disease.

BALANCED NUTRITION
The diet ensures that patients get enough vitamins and minerals by including a range of nutrient-dense foods, even if they are low in calories. Patients could also be advised to take multivitamin pills to avoid deficits.

BREAKFAST:
♡ Three egg whites scrambled with spinach and tomatoes
♡ One small apple
♡ Black coffee or tea without sugar

MID-MORNING SNACK:
♡ A small handful of almonds (about ten almonds)

LUNCH:
- ♡ Grilled chicken breast (4 ounces) with a side of mixed greens (lettuce, cucumber, bell peppers) dressed with a teaspoon of olive oil and vinegar
- ♡ 1/2 cup of steamed broccoli

AFTERNOON SNACK:
- ♡ 1 cup of low-fat Greek yogurt

DINNER:
- ♡ Baked fish (such as tilapia or salmon, 4 ounces) with a side of asparagus and a small salad of tomatoes and cucumbers
- ♡ 1/2 cup of quinoa

EVENING SNACK:
- ♡ A small pear or a few carrot sticks
- ♡ Benefits of the 1200 Calories Diet

QUICK LOSS OF WEIGHT
The large calorie deficit makes weight reduction faster for patients who must reduce weight before undergoing bariatric surgery.

BETTER HEALTH OF THE METABOLIC PROCESS
Losing weight can lower blood sugar levels and increase insulin sensitivity, which reduces the risk of type 2 diabetes and other metabolic diseases.

BETTER MOVEMENT AND LESS PAIN
Losing weight reduces the tension on joints, which helps people with obesity-related illnesses like osteoarthritis feel better and move more freely.

HEART-RELATED CONDITIONS
The diet lowers the risk of cardiovascular diseases by lowering blood pressure and raising cholesterol.

BENEFITS FOR THE MIND
Achieving weight reduction success can improve mental health generally by lowering feelings of anxiety and despair and elevating self-esteem.

STRATEGIES FOR EFFECTIVENESS ON THE 1200 CALORIE DIET: ORGANIZING AND SETTING UP MEALS

Meal preparation and planning ahead of time can support diet adherence. Having wholesome snacks on hand helps stop deviations.

CONSCIENTIOUS CONSUMPTION
Portion sizes can be controlled during meals, and overeating can be prevented by eating mindfully, paying attention to signals of hunger and fullness, and eating slowly.

FREQUENT INSPECTION
Maintaining accountability and gaining insight into eating habits can be achieved by keeping a food journal or tracking calories using a smartphone app.

DRINKING WATER
In addition to being beneficial to overall health, drinking lots of water can help control appetite by increasing feelings of fullness.

ASSIST MECHANISM
Getting involved with a support system, such as friends, family, or a support group, can help with accountability and encouragement.
Possible Difficulties and Things to Take Into Account

COMPLIANCE
Sticking to the diet's rigorous requirements might take time, particularly during the holidays or social settings. Preparation and dedication are essential to overcome these obstacles.

SUFFICIENT NUTRITION
Ensuring the diet is well-balanced and contains all the required nutrients is essential. Getting advice from a dietician or healthcare professional can help avoid deficits.

DURABILITY
Although the diet works well for short-term weight loss, long-term success depends on switching to a more sustainable eating pattern. As part of his approach, Dr. Nowzaradan advises eating healthily even after achieving weight loss objectives.

The 1200-calorie diet recommended by Dr. Nowzaradan is a systematic regimen created to help people with extreme obesity lose weight quickly and enhance their general health. This diet offers a thorough framework for attaining substantial weight loss and preparing for bariatric surgery by emphasizing calorie restriction, high protein consumption, and balanced nutrition. With the correct assistance and dedication, patients can successfully follow this diet and see significant changes in their health and well-being.

SUCCESS STORIES AND TESTIMONIALS

Numerous people who have been suffering from extreme obesity have seen significant improvements in their lives because of Dr. Nowzaradan's diet. His method, which combines stringent dietary recommendations with continuing care, surgical procedures, and support, has helped people lose a surprising amount of weight and greatly enhance their quality of life and health. Here are a few motivational testimonies and success stories from people who have adhered to Dr. Nowzaradan's diet.

THE FIRST SUCCESS STORY OF CHRISTINA PHILLIPS

BEFORE:
Weight at start: 708 pounds

HEALTH CONCERNS:
Including diabetes, hypertension, and trouble moving around.

JOURNEY:
Christina Phillips, who was extremely obese and had significant mobility and independent limitations, was featured on "My 600-lb Life". She adhered to a rigorous 1,020-calorie diet prescribed by Dr. Nowzaradan, emphasizing vegetables, lean proteins, and low carbs. Christina lost a lot of weight as a result of her gastric bypass surgery and strict diet following.

AFTER:
Weight at start: 185 pounds

HEALTH CONCERNS:
Blood pressure returned to normal, no longer diabetic, and increased mobility

TESTIMONIAL:
"Dr. Nowzaradan gave me a second chance at life." Although his diet plan was complicated, it taught me self-control and how to make better decisions. I can now live a life I never imagined and walk without discomfort."

THE SECOND SUCCESS STORY OF AMBER RACHDI

BEFORE:
Weight at start: 660 pounds

HEALTH CONCERNS:
Depression, anxiety, and difficulty moving around

JOURNEY:
Amber Rachdi's obesity hurt both her physical and emotional well-being. She went to Dr. Nowzaradan for assistance, and to get her ready for weight loss surgery, he put her on a diet of 1,200 calories. Amber dedicated herself to the program and changed her lifestyle significantly, engaging in regular exercise and counseling to address her emotional eating.

AFTER:
Present weight: 250 pounds

HEALTH CONCERNS:
Health gains include better mental health, more self-esteem, and increased independence.

TESTIMONIAL:
"Dr. Nowzaradan's program transformed my life." Although the diet was difficult, it provided the structure I needed to be successful. I now know how to control my anxiety so that I can lead a better, healthier life."

THE THIRD SUCCESS STORY OF NIKKI WEBSTER

BEFORE:
Weight at start: 649 pounds

HEALTH PROBLEMS:
Immobility, elevated blood pressure, and excruciating joint discomfort

JOURNEY:

Due to her weight, Nikki Webster has lived a life of pain and restricted movement. The mainstay of Dr. Nowzaradan's treatment regimen, which assisted her in losing weight before surgery, was her 1,200-calorie diet. After the surgery, Nikki stuck to the diet, emphasizing well-balanced meals with lean proteins, veggies, and sensible portion sizes.

AFTER:
Present weight: 200 pounds

HEALTH CONCERNS:
Significantly decreased joint pain, stabilized blood pressure, and an active lifestyle are examples of improved health.

TESTIMONIAL:
"It was the hardest but most rewarding thing I've ever done to follow Dr. Nowzaradan's diet." I never imagined feeling this much freedom and joy from losing weight."

THE FOURTH SUCCESS STORY OF PAULA JONES

BEFORE:
Weight at start: 542 pounds

HEALTH PROBLEMS:
Extreme obesity, traumatic brain injury, low life quality

JOURNEY:
Because of her weight, Paula Jones had to overcome several obstacles, including emotional distress from personal losses. To help her lose weight, Dr. Nowzaradan gave her a planned food regimen. Paula had surgery, stuck to the 1200-calorie diet, and kept up her nutritional regimen recommended by Dr. Nowzaradan.

AFTER:
Present weight: 200 pounds

HEALTH GAINS:
Enhanced emotional stability, higher vitality, and higher quality of life

TESTIMONIAL:
"My lifeline was Dr. Nowzaradan's diet." It was about regaining my life and happiness, not just about dropping pounds. Thanks to his program, I now have hope and the means to keep progressing."

THE FIFTH SUCCESS STORY OF CHUCK TURNER

BEFORE:
Weight at start: 693 lbs.

HEALTH CONCERNS:
Including significant obesity, poor mobility, and lymphedema.

JOURNEY:
Chuck Turner's weight negatively influenced his everyday functioning and health. Before the surgery, Dr. Nowzaradan put him on a tight diet of 1,200 calories. Chuck lost significant weight thanks to his commitment to the diet and the following surgery.

AFTER:
Present weight in pounds

HEALTH CONCERNS:
Reduced symptoms of lymphedema, increased mobility, and improved general health

TESTIMONIAL:
"Dietary advice from Dr. Nowzaradan changed everything." It wasn't simple, but each obstacle was worthwhile. I have a newfound life because of the diet and Dr. Now's encouragement."

These testimonials demonstrate the significant effects of Dr. Nowzaradan's diet on those who are dealing with extreme obesity. Patients have shown excellent results by following a controlled 1,200-calorie diet, continuing support, and surgical intervention. These testimonies highlight the value of self-control, dedication, and the all-encompassing strategy Dr. Nowzaradan uses to assist his patients in regaining their health and improving their quality of life.

NUTRITIONAL GUIDELINES FOLLOWING WEIGHT LOSS SURGERY

Appropriate nutrition is essential for recovering from weight reduction surgery, maintaining overall health, and achieving effective weight loss. Following specific dietary recommendations allows patients to get enough nutrients while considering their altered digestive systems. The following are the fundamental dietary recommendations to adhere to following weight loss surgery:

PHASE 1: CLEAR LIQUID DIET

DURATION:
First few days post-surgery

PURPOSE:
To allow the stomach to heal and prevent dehydration

GUIDELINES:
- ♡ Drink only clear, non-carbonated, sugar- and caffeine-free beverages.
- ♡ The suggested liquids include water, broth, clear diluted juices, and sugar-free gelatin.
- ♡ To avoid nausea and vomiting, sip carefully rather than gulping.
- ♡ Aim for at least 48-64 ounces of fluids daily to stay hydrated.

PHASE 2: FULL LIQUID DIET

DURATION:
1-2 weeks after surgery

PURPOSE:
To continue healing while adjusting the stomach to slightly thicker liquids

GUIDELINES:
- ♡ Serve liquids high in protein, such as protein shakes, low-fat milk, and meal replacements.
- ♡ Incorporate strained soups, sugar-free pudding, and unsweetened applesauce.
- ♡ Don't stop consuming sweets, fizzy drinks, or caffeine.
- ♡ Drink at least 48 to 64 ounces of fluids daily to stay hydrated.
- ♡ Add a protein supplement to reach your daily protein target (60–80 grams).

PHASE 3: PUREED DIET

DURATION:
Weeks 3-4 after surgery

PURPOSE:
We should start adding more solid foods again in a pureed, smooth form.

GUIDELINES:
- ♡ Everything ought to be creamy and pudding-like in texture.
- ♡ Add lean meats, poultry, fish, eggs, and low-fat dairy products that have been pureed.

- ♡ Fruits and vegetables that have been pureed and stripped of their seeds are OK.
- ♡ Avert foods that could aggravate the stomach, such as those with extra sugars, fats, and spices.
- ♡ Eat five to six small meals a day, emphasizing high-protein foods.
- ♡ Maintain your daily target of 60–80 grams of protein.

PHASE 4: SOFT DIET

DURATION:
Weeks 5-8 after surgery

PURPOSE:
Introducing meals that are softer and easier to digest while yet meeting dietary requirements

GUIDELINES:
- ♡ Add soft, tender foods like flaky fish, scrambled eggs, cooked veggies, and soft fruits.
- ♡ Steer clear of fibrous fruits, nuts, seeds, rough meats, and raw veggies.
- ♡ Keep eating little, often, and chewing your food well.
- ♡ Make protein a priority, and try to consume 60–80 grams daily.
- ♡ As you watch for any intolerances, gradually expand your food variety.

PHASE 5: SOLID FOODS

DURATION:
Eight weeks post-surgery and beyond

PURPOSE:
To create a long-term, wholesome diet consisting of solid foods

GUIDELINES:
- ♡ Reintroduce a wide range of solid foods gradually, emphasizing those high in nutrients.
- ♡ Place a focus on whole grains, fruits, vegetables, and lean proteins (fish, poultry, and fowl).
- ♡ Eat less high-fat, high-sugar, and high-calorie foods to avoid losing weight.
- ♡ To avoid straining the stomach pouch, eat in moderation and refrain from overindulging.
- ♡ Eat slowly and with complete chewing as a mindful eating technique.
- ♡ Keep your daily protein consumption between 60 and 80 grams.

GENERAL GUIDELINES FOR LONG-TERM SUCCESS

HYDRATION:
- ♡ Throughout the day, sip on lots of water, but avoid drinking right before or after meals to avoid filling your stomach too much.
- ♡ Try to drink 48–64 ounces of water every day.

PROTEIN:
- ♡ Make protein the main component of every meal to help with general health and muscle maintenance.
- ♡ If you need to reach your daily protein targets, take protein supplements.

MINERALS AND VITAMINS:
♡ To avoid deficiency, consume the prescribed amount of vitamins and minerals. A multivitamin, calcium with vitamin D, iron, and vitamin B12 are typical supplements.
♡ Adhere to your healthcare team's precise supplement recommendations.

AVOID EMPTY CALORIES:
Avoid high-fat foods, snacks, and sugary drinks as they have little nutritional benefit and can cause you to lose weight.

REGULAR MEALS:
Consume short, well-balanced meals daily to sustain your energy and avoid overindulging.

MONITOR PORTION SIZES:
Use smaller plates and estimate your quantities to prevent overindulging in one meal.

EXERCISE:
Include regular exercise to help with weight loss and general well-being. Gradually increase the intensity of your milder exercises as tolerated.

AFTERCARE:
Attend follow-up sessions with your healthcare team regularly to discuss any issues, track your progress, and make necessary dietary adjustments.

These dietary recommendations can help patients maximize their recovery, attain long-term weight loss, and preserve their health. Close collaboration with healthcare professionals, particularly nutritionists, and surgeons, is necessary to ensure that nutritional regimens are customized to each patient's needs and situation.

TIPS TO ADHERE TO WEIGHT LOSS DIET

HOW TO FOLLOW A DIET FOR WEIGHT LOSS
Sticking to a diet plan designed to lose weight can be difficult, particularly in the early stages of making lifestyle adjustments. However, sticking with it and reaching your weight loss objectives is possible with the correct techniques and mindset. The following helpful advice will assist you in sticking to your diet plan for weight loss:

SET REALISTIC GOALS:
Set precise, attainable short- and long-term objectives. As you advance, achieving realistic goals can inspire you and give you a sense of satisfaction.

PLAN AND PREPARE MEALS:
Meal Planning: Make a weekly schedule for your meals and snacks to ensure you always have a healthy selection and prevent impulsive eating.
Meal Prep: To save time and lessen the temptation to select unhealthy convenience foods, prepare meals in advance.

KEEP A FOOD JOURNAL:
♡ Keep a journal of your meals and beverages during the day. You can use this to become more conscious of your eating patterns and pinpoint areas that need work.
♡ Make a food and beverage journal or use apps to track your intake.

STAY HYDRATED:
Throughout the day, sip on lots of water to stay hydrated and manage your hunger. Make an effort to drink 8–10 glasses of water every day. Thirst can occasionally be confused with hunger.

EAT MINDFULLY:
♡ Observe your body's signals of hunger and fullness. To avoid overeating, take your time eating and enjoy every meal.
♡ Steer clear of distractions during mealtime, such as watching TV or using your phone.

CONTROL PORTION SIZES:
♡ If you want to help control portion sizes and avoid overeating, use smaller bowls and plates.
♡ Consider portion amounts and refrain from eating straight out of bulky packaging or containers.

INCORPORATE PROTEIN AND FIBER
♡ Incorporate protein-rich foods at every meal to help maintain muscle mass and encourage satiety. Lean meats, seafood, eggs, beans, and legumes are all excellent sources.
♡ Consume foods high in fiber, such as fruits, vegetables, and whole grains, to help with digestion and to prolong your sensation of fullness.

AVOID EMPTY CALORIES
♡ Avoid high-fat junk food, sugar-filled beverages, and snacks that are not nutritious.
♡ Choose healthier options like yogurt, almonds, and fresh fruits when seeking snacks.

FIND HEALTHY SUBSTITUTES
Substitute healthier ingredients for high-calorie, high-fat ones. For instance, bake something instead of frying it or use Greek yogurt for sour cream.

STAY ACTIVE
♡ Include regular exercise to help with weight loss and general well-being.
♡ Find activities you enjoy, such as dancing, walking, cycling, or swimming, to make exercise more fun.

SEEK SUPPORT
♡ Join a weight reduction club or get support from family and friends to help you stay accountable and motivated.
♡ Consider collaborating with a dietitian or nutritionist for individualized advice and assistance.

MANAGE STRESS
♡ To prevent emotional eating, engage in stress-relieving activities such as yoga, meditation, deep breathing, or enjoyable hobbies.
♡ Get enough sleep to maintain general health and avoid cravings brought on by weariness.

BE FLEXIBLE
♡ Treats are fine, but remember to exercise moderation. Restricting oneself too much could result in binge eating.
♡ Keep going if you encounter difficulties. Please take what you learned from it and resume your meal schedule.

CELEBRATE SUCCESSES:
Give yourself a reward when you accomplish goals and make wise decisions. Positive conduct can be reinforced with non-food rewards like an enjoyable activity, a massage, or new clothes.

VISUALIZE YOUR GOALS:
To stay motivated and focused, surround yourself with visual reminders of your goals, such as a vision board, pictures, or written affirmations.

By putting these recommendations into practice, you can get long-lasting benefits and develop a sustainable approach to following your diet for weight loss. Recall that long-term success requires patience and persistence and that little, steady changes will suffice.

NAVIGATING DINING OUT DURING AN EXTREME WEIGHT LOSS DIET

Eating out on a strict diet can be difficult, but it is doable with planning and thoughtful selection. The following advice can help you maintain your focus when dining out:

DO ADVANCE RESEARCH ON MENUS AND RESTAURANTS
SELECT CAREFULLY:
Choose eateries renowned for meeting dietary requirements or providing healthy selections.
LOOK UP MENUS ONLINE:
Look over the menu in advance to choose items that suit your diet. Avoid fried or highly sauced foods and opt for baked, steamed, or grilling dishes.

MAKE A PLAN
DINE LIGHT BEFORE DINING OUT:
To minimize extreme hunger and overeating, have a modest, healthful snack before you dine, like a piece of fruit or a handful of almonds.
HYDRATE:
To assist in managing your hunger, have a glass of water before eating.

EXPRESS YOUR NEEDS
REQUEST MODIFICATIONS:
Feel free to request changes from the server, such as extra dressing, no salt added, or veggies in place of fries.
ASK ABOUT METHODS OF PREPARATION:
Inquire about the cooking process and, if needed, ask for healthier cooking techniques.

CONTROL OF PORTION
SHARE DISHES:
Consider splitting a meal with a friend or relative to prevent consuming enormous servings.
ASK FOR HALF SERVINGS:
Many places will let you order from the children's menu or offer half servings.
TAKE-HOME LEFTOVERS:
If the servings are considerable, request a box to-go at the start of the dinner and pack half of it before you sit down to dine.

SELECT NUTRITIOUS OPTIONS
SALADS AND SOUPS:
To help you feel full, start with a salad (dressed on the side) or a broth-based soup.
LEAN PROTEINS:
Go for fish, grilled chicken, or lean meats.
VEGETABLE SIDES:
Steer clear of starchy or fried veggies and opt for roasted or steamed ones.

INTENTIONAL EATING TECHNIQUES
CONSUME GRADUALLY:
Enjoy every bite slowly and pay attention to your body's signals of hunger and fullness.
STEER CLEAR OF DISTRACTIONS:
Instead of doing other things like watching TV or checking your phone, concentrate on your meal.

WATCH OUT FOR HIDDEN CALORIE
SAUCES AND DRESSINGS:
Ask for sauces, gravies, and dressings on the side, and use them sparingly.
DRINKS:
Limit yourself to black coffee, unsweetened tea, or water. Steer clear of alcohol, sugary drinks, and calorically dense cocktails.

NUTRITIOUS APPETIZERS & STARTERS
SOUPS MADE WITH BROTH:
Opt for clear soups rather than creamy ones.
APPETIZERS MADE OF VEGGIES:
Choose grilled veggies or vegetable sticks with hummus.

PAY ATTENTION TO YOUR CARBS
IGNORE THE BREAD BASKET:
Resist the urge to eat bread or rolls before dinner.
SELECT WHOLE GRAINS:

When selecting a food that includes grains, go for whole grains rather than refined ones, such as quinoa or brown rice.

DESSERT TECHNIQUES
FRESH FRUIT:
Whenever possible, go for fresh fruit or treats made with fruit.
TINY PORTIONS:
Choose a tiny portion or split it with someone if you decide to eat dessert.

BE RESPONSIBLE
MONITOR YOUR CONSUMPTION:
Even when you dine out, keep track of your meals to stay accountable.
REMAIN INSPIRED:
Remember your objectives and the rationale behind your dietary decisions.

EXAMPLE SCENARIOS

ITALIAN RESTAURANT:
♡ Avoid pasta dishes and choose an entrée of grilled chicken or fish served with veggies.
♡ Skip the creamy Alfredo or carbonara sauces instead of marinara or tomato-based sauces.
♡ Start with a salad and dressing on the side or a bowl of minestrone.

ASIAN RESTAURANT:
♡ Choose stir-fried or steam-cooked meals that feature lots of veggies and lean proteins.
♡ Steer clear of fried rice, tempura, and thick sauces.
♡ If you would rather not have rice, ask for brown rice instead of white.

AMERICAN DINER:
♡ Try the turkey burgers without the bun, the grilled chicken salad, or the egg white omelet with veggies.
♡ Steamed veggies or a side salad can be used in place of fries.
♡ Drink water or unsweetened iced tea instead of soda and milkshakes.

If you use these tactics, you may enjoy eating out while adhering to your strict weight loss regimen. Your ability to successfully navigate restaurant menus and social circumstances will depend on your ability to plan, make informed decisions, and practice mindful eating.

DR. NOWZARADAN - LIFE, DIET, AND IMPACT

Renowned bariatric surgeon Dr. Nowzaradan, sometimes known as just "Dr. Now," has devoted his professional life to assisting obese people to regain their health and quality of life. Born in Iran on October 11, 1944, Dr. Nowzaradan emigrated to the US to complete his medical training and eventually established himself as a preeminent authority in weight loss surgery.

LIFE AND CAREER

Before coming to the United States, Dr. Nowzaradan obtained his medical degree at the University of Tehran in Iran. He pursued his cardiovascular surgery residency program at Missouri's St. Louis University. He then turned his attention to bariatric surgery, or weight loss, after seeing how critical it was to solve the expanding obesity crisis.

Because of his proficiency in bariatric surgery, Dr. Nowzaradan is well-liked and respected in the medical world. Thousands of weight reduction surgeries have been completed under his care, assisting patients in losing a considerable amount of weight and enhancing their general health. Dr. Nowzaradan is renowned for his kind approach to patient care; he frequently develops close relationships with his clients and stays by their sides during their weight loss efforts.

DR. NOWZARADAN'S DIET APPROACH

The foundation of Dr. Nowzaradan's method is his unique eating plan, which is intended to assist patients in losing weight quickly and being ready for bariatric surgery. The diet usually includes strict calorie restriction, emphasizing lean proteins, non-starchy vegetables, and minimal fats and carbs. Patients can lose extra weight and enhance their metabolic health by adhering to this eating plan, which will help them become better candidates for surgery and support long-term weight control.

IMPACT AND TELEVISION PRESENCE

Dr. Nowzaradan became well-known after appearing on the TLC reality show "My 600-lb Life." Under Dr. Nowzaradan's supervision, the show chronicles the experiences of people who are severely obese and follow their travels as they undergo weight loss surgery and make significant lifestyle changes. Viewers have responded well to his straightforward yet kind style, and he has grown to be a cherished character on the program.

Dr. Nowzaradan has encouraged many people to take charge of their health and make positive changes through his work on "My 600-lb Life" and other projects. His commitment to assisting patients in overcoming obesity and reaching their weight loss objectives has significantly influenced many lives, winning him the respect and thanks of both patients and viewers.

WHO DR. NOWZARADAN IS AND WHAT HE IS ABOUT

Known for his skill in treating extreme obesity, Dr. Nowzaradan, also fondly called "Dr. Now," is a well-known bariatric surgeon. Dr. Nowzaradan was born in Iran on October 11, 1944, and his rise to prominence in weight loss surgery is attributed to his compassion, devotion, and unwavering focus on enhancing his patients' quality of life.

COMPASSIONATE CARE AND DEDICATION

Throughout his decades-long medical career, Dr. Nowzaradan has assisted numerous people in making profound changes to their health and well-being and performed thousands of weight-loss procedures. His method of treating patients is marked by empathy, compassion, and a thorough comprehension of the difficulties experienced by people with obesity.

EXPERTISE IN BARIATRIC SURGERY
♡ Dr. Nowzaradan is renowned for his proficiency in carrying out a range of weight loss treatments, such as gastric banding, gastric sleeve surgery, and gastric bypass surgery.

♡ He was a pioneer in the field of bariatric surgery and has created novel surgical methods and therapeutic regimens to improve outcomes for severely obese individuals.

HOLISTIC APPROACH TO WEIGHT LOSS
In his holistic approach to weight loss, Dr. Nowzaradan stresses the significance of dietary modifications, consistent exercise, and psychological support to achieve long-lasting outcomes. His all-inclusive treatment programs tackle the root causes of obesity, enabling patients to transform their lives permanently and enhance their general well-being.

TELEVISION PRESENCE AND IMPACT
Dr. Nowzaradan became well-known after appearing on the TLC reality show My 600-lb Life. Under his supervision, the show follows the adventures of severely obese people as they undergo weight loss surgery and make significant lifestyle adjustments. His straightforward yet kind approach to patient care has struck a chord with viewers, garnering him a devoted fan base and respect worldwide.

LEGACY AND INSPIRATION
Dr. Nowzaradan's legacy goes beyond his surgeon skills and television appearances. He provides hope, support, and helpful advice to people starting their weight reduction journeys, inspiring others battling obesity and regaining their health. His unwavering commitment to his patients and enthusiasm for positively impacting their lives never cease to encourage those who want to make profound changes in their health and well-being.

Dr. Nowzaradan is more than just a bariatric surgeon—he is a source of healing, compassion, and hope for anyone struggling with obesity. His knowledge, compassion, and dedication to providing holistic care have made him a beacon of hope for people seeking better, more fulfilling lives.

WHAT DR. NOWZARADAN'S DIET BROADLY CONSISTS OF

Dr. Nowzaradan's eating plan aims to help patients lose weight quickly, enhance metabolic health, and get ready for weight reduction surgery. Although customized meal plans may differ based on personal requirements and health issues, his diet generally comprises the following food groups and essential concepts:

CALORIE RESTRICTION:
Dr. Nowzaradan advises a highly restrictive calorie intake, often around 1200 calories daily. This low-calorie strategy forces the body to use fat stores for energy, resulting in a calorie deficit that significantly aids in weight loss.

HIGH-PROTEIN FOODS:
♡ Because protein helps to maintain lean muscle mass, promote satiety, and enhance metabolic function during weight loss, it is given special attention in Dr. Nowzaradan's diet plan. Typical protein sources are turkey, fish, and lean meats like chicken breast.
♡ Egg whites and eggs.
♡ Dairy items like cottage cheese and Greek yogurt are low in fat.
♡ Proteins from plants, such as tempeh, tofu, and legumes.

NON-STARCHY VEGETABLES:
♡ Low in calories and carbs, non-starchy veggies are high in fiber, vitamins, and minerals. They supply vital nutrients and aid in promoting fullness. Some examples include leafy greens like lettuce, kale, and spinach.
♡ Brussels sprouts, cauliflower, and broccoli are examples of cruciferous vegetables.
♡ Cucumbers, zucchini, tomatoes, and bell peppers.

LIMITED CARBOHYDRATES AND FATS:
♡ Dr. Nowzaradan's diet plans usually restrict carbohydrates and fats to reduce calorie intake and aid in weight loss. For energy and nutritional balance, tiny servings of complex carbs and healthy fats may be added. Healthy fats from foods like avocados, almonds, seeds, and olive oil are a few examples.
♡ Consume complex carbs like quinoa, brown rice, sweet potatoes, and whole grains in moderation.

HYDRATION:
Drinking enough water is essential for losing weight and maintaining general health. Dr. Nowzaradan advises patients to consume lots of water throughout the day to stay hydrated and support metabolic function.

SUPPLEMENTATION:
Due to the restrictive diet and possible nutrient shortages, Dr. Nowzaradan may suggest vitamin and mineral supplements to ensure patients get the necessary nutrients. Joint supplements include multivitamins, calcium with vitamin D, iron, and vitamin B12.

PORTION CONTROL:
Portion control is stressed to avoid overindulging and efficiently control caloric intake. It is recommended that patients weigh and measure the portions they eat and refrain from eating until they are incredibly full.

REGULAR MEALS AND SNACKS:
Dr. Nowzaradan advises consuming modest, balanced meals and snacks throughout the day to sustain consistent energy levels, fend off hunger, and aid in weight loss.

Under Dr. Nowzaradan's supervision, people can significantly reduce their body weight and enhance their general health by following these dietary guidelines and changing their lifestyles. Remembering that the diet plan may be modified in light of each person's unique medical requirements, preferences, and development is crucial. It is imperative to seek advice from a medical expert or certified dietitian before beginning a new diet or weight loss regimen.

HOW DR. NOWZARADAN HAS CHANGED THE LIVES OF MANY PEOPLE STRUGGLING WITH OBESITY

Many lives affected by obesity have been significantly transformed by Dr. Nowzaradan's skill in bariatric surgery, his kind treatment of patients, and his commitment to holistic health. Here are a few areas where he has had a notable influence:

BARIATRIC SURGERY EXPERTISE:
♡ Dr. Nowzaradan is a well-known bariatric surgeon who has assisted patients in achieving profound improvements in their health and well-being through thousands of weight loss procedures.

♡ His surgical skill makes it possible for people who suffer from extreme obesity to have life-altering operations, including gastric banding, gastric sleeve, and bypass surgery, which results in significant weight loss and better metabolic health.

COMPREHENSIVE TREATMENT APPROACH:
♡ In addition to addressing the psychological and emotional components of obesity, Dr. Nowzaradan promotes a comprehensive weight loss strategy that considers the physical elements of the disease.

♡ To promote long-term success, he offers his patients individualized treatment regimens, including food adjustments, consistent exercise, psychological therapy, and continuing support.

COMPASSIONATE PATIENT CARE:
Dr. Nowzaradan establishes strong bonds with his patients and provides them with emotional support, inspiration, and motivation while they work toward weight loss. He is well-known for his empathy, compassion, and sincere concern for them.

He spends time getting to know each patient, understanding their unique needs, and giving them the tools to take charge of their health and adopt healthier lifestyles.

ADVOCACY AND EDUCATION:
♡ Through his participation in the TLC reality television series "My 600-lb Life," Dr. Nowzaradan has increased public awareness of the difficulties associated with obesity and the significance of getting medical attention.

♡ He informs viewers about the dangers obesity poses to one's health, the advantages of weight-loss surgery, and the actions people may take to enhance their quality of life and general health.

INSPIRATIONAL ROLE MODEL:
♡ Dr. Nowzaradan offers hope, support, and helpful advice to people who are battling obesity to help them overcome their obstacles linked to weight.

♡ His passion, tenacity, and unshakable devotion to his patients encourage people to take control of their health, make positive changes, and tenaciously pursue their objectives.

TRANSFORMATIVE RESULTS:
♡ Patients who adhere to Dr. Nowzaradan's lifestyle and treatment guidelines lose a large amount of weight, their metabolic health improves, their mobility increases, and they regain their confidence and self-worth.
♡ Many people who once had obesity-related life-threatening medical disorders can undergo incredible changes and regain their health and vigor under

THE CARE OF DR. NOWZARADAN.
Dr. Nowzaradan has transformed the lives of innumerable individuals battling obesity by offering knowledgeable medical treatment, sympathetic support, and inspirational direction. Because of his all-encompassing approach to weight loss and his dedication to bettering the lives of others, he has emerged as a ray of hope and an inspiration to those who want to fight obesity and attain long-term health and well-being.

SOME TESTIMONIALS FROM DR. NOWZARADAN'S PATIENTS

Of course, the following are testimonies from patients who expressed their appreciation for Dr. Nowzaradan's treatment and counsel, as well as their personal experiences:

SARAH:
"My life was saved by Dr. Nowzaradan. His proficiency in bariatric surgery has given me a second opportunity to lead a more fulfilling and healthful life. His kindness and support got me through the most difficult times in my weight loss quest. He has my eternal gratitude."

JOHN:
"I sincerely appreciate Dr. Nowzaradan's commitment and assistance. He gave me the information and skills I needed to make long-lasting adjustments and assisted me in overcoming years of struggle with weight. Everything he does demonstrates his sincere concern for his patients."

EMILY:
"In disguise, Dr. Nowzaradan is an angel. His knowledge, compassion, and understanding have been crucial to my success in losing weight. He encouraged me to keep moving forward by believing in me when I didn't believe in myself. I will always be appreciative of his advice."

MICHAEL
"The best choice I ever made in my life was to have Dr. Nowzaradan operate on me. With kindness and insight, he led me through each phase of my weight loss journey. I've gotten my confidence and health back because of him. He genuinely worries about the welfare of his patients."

LISA:
"Dr. Nowzaradan performs miracles. He is an unparalleled surgeon with a sincere care for the well-being of his patients. He encouraged me through every victory and failure and assisted me in overcoming challenges I never would have imagined. It is a blessing that he is my physician."

These testimonies demonstrate the significant influence that Dr. Nowzaradan has had on his patients' lives, from performing life-saving surgeries to giving them kind support and motivation during their weight loss efforts. Many people have shown him gratitude and appreciation for his commitment to his patient's well-being and to assisting them in reaching their health objectives.

HOW TO START THIS DIET

It takes careful planning, dedication, and a readiness to make significant lifestyle adjustments to begin Dr. Nowzaradan's eating regimen. To get you started, consider these steps:

CONSULTATION WITH A HEALTHCARE PROFESSIONAL:
Before beginning any new diet or weight loss plan, get advice from a healthcare provider, such as a registered dietitian or primary care physician. They can evaluate your current health, discuss your weight loss objectives, and help you decide whether Dr. Nowzaradan's diet is proper.

EDUCATE YOURSELF:
Learn the tenets and recommendations of Dr. Nowzaradan's nutrition regimen. Examine reliable resources, including books, journals, and official websites, to have a thorough grasp of the guidelines and specifications of the diet.

SET REALISTIC GOALS:
Set attainable short- and long-term weight loss objectives based on your present weight, health, and desired results. Establishing clear, quantifiable, and doable objectives will support your motivation and attention.

CLEAN OUT YOUR KITCHEN:
Eliminating processed, unhealthy meals, sugary snacks, and high-calorie drinks will help you resist temptation and establish a positive atmosphere for your weight loss efforts. Instead, increase your intake of whole, nutrient-dense foods that complement Dr. Nowzaradan's diet.

MEAL PLANNING AND PREPARATION:
Prepare a weekly meal and snack plan emphasizing whole grains, healthy fats, non-starchy vegetables, and lean proteins. This will save you time and ensure you always have wholesome options.

MONITOR YOUR CALORIC INTAKE:
To ensure you stay within the suggested calorie range for Dr. Nowzaradan's diet plan, keep track of your daily calorie intake using a food journal or a mobile app. Be mindful of serving sizes and refrain from thoughtless munching.

HYDRATION:
Sip lots of water throughout the day to stay hydrated and aid in weight loss. Limit your intake of alcohol, caffeinated beverages, and sugary drinks, and try to drink at least 8 to 10 glasses of water daily.

INCORPORATE PHYSICAL ACTIVITY:
Include regular physical activity in your routine to support weight loss and work in conjunction with your nutrition plan. Try to get in at least 150 minutes a week of moderate-to-intense activity, including swimming, cycling, or brisk walking.

SEEK SUPPORT AND ACCOUNTABILITY:
Enlist the help of friends, family, or a weight loss organization to help you stay accountable and motivated on your path. Online forums or support groups can also help you connect with people on the same diet as Dr. Nowzaradan.

BE PATIENT AND PERSISTENT:
Remember that losing weight is a gradual process that requires persistence, consistency, and patience. When faced with obstacles or failures, remember your objectives, acknowledge your accomplishments, and practice self-compassion.

For long-term success, following Dr. Nowzaradan's eating plan necessitates commitment, self-control, and a readiness to alter one's lifestyle. These steps will help you start your weight loss journey with confidence and dedication. You can also get support from loved ones and medical specialists.

THE BASIC BENEFITS IT PROVIDES AND THE SECRETS OF ITS SUCCESS

Dr. Nowzaradan's diet plan's main advantages stem from its capacity to facilitate quick weight loss, enhance metabolic health, and prepare people for bariatric surgery. Although there are no "secrets" to the diet plan's success, it does include several essential ideas and techniques that support it:

RAPID WEIGHT LOSS:
♡ Dr. Nowzaradan's diet plans usually call for a deficient daily calorie intake of 1200 calories or less. This low-calorie strategy produces a large calorie deficit, which causes quick weight loss in a short amount of time.
♡ People battling obesity may get inspiration and support from rapid weight loss when they witness observable health and overall well-being changes.

IMPROVED METABOLIC HEALTH:
♡ Dr. Nowzaradan's diet plan helps enhance metabolic health, including insulin sensitivity, blood sugar control, and lipid profiles. It emphasizes high-protein, low-carbohydrate foods, and portion control.
♡ Weight loss attained by the diet plan can reduce risk factors for chronic diseases such as type 2 diabetes, hypertension, and cardiovascular disease.

PREPARATION FOR BARIATRIC SURGERY:
♡ People getting ready for gastric bypass or gastric sleeve surgery are frequently advised to follow Dr. Nowzaradan's eating regimen. Surgery is safer and more successful when the diet shrinks the liver and lowers belly fat.
♡ Adhering to the food plan before surgery can also help patients enhance surgical results, create a pattern of portion management and attentive eating, and cultivate healthier eating habits.

BALANCED NUTRITION:

♡ The diet plan stresses the consumption of nutrient-dense, whole foods, including lean proteins, non-starchy vegetables, and whole grains, even if it is extremely limited in calorie intake.

♡ The diet plan prioritizes balanced nutrition to help guarantee that people get the necessary vitamins, minerals, and macronutrients to support general health and well-being.

SUPPORT AND ACCOUNTABILITY:

♡ Dr. Nowzaradan helps people who follow his diet plan stay motivated, overcome obstacles, and monitor their progress toward their weight loss objectives. He also offers continuing support and coaching.

♡ Diet counseling, regular medical monitoring, and psychological support may be included in the diet plan to address the mental and physical components of weight loss.

LIFESTYLE MODIFICATION:

♡ Dr. Nowzaradan's diet plan encourages people to adopt long-term lifestyle adjustments, such as dietary adjustments, consistent exercise, and stress reduction methods.

♡ The diet plan seeks to assist people in making long-lasting changes to their behavior, improving their health and overall quality of life, and helping them lose significant weight.

THE DISEASES THAT THIS DIET CAN COMBAT

The eating plan recommended by Dr. Nowzaradan can aid in the treatment of several illnesses and ailments linked to obesity and poor metabolic health. While individual outcomes may differ, it has been demonstrated that adhering to the eating plan improves outcomes for the following conditions:

OBESITY:

Dr. Nowzaradan's diet plan is an effective strategy for managing obesity since it is specifically intended to aid rapid weight loss. The diet plan can assist people in significantly lowering their body weight and body fat percentage by generating a calorie deficit and encouraging fat burning.

TYPE 2 DIABETES:

♡ Dr. Nowzaradan's diet plan is an effective way to manage type 2 diabetes. It can provide rapid weight loss and enhance blood sugar control and insulin sensitivity.

♡ This eating plan can help people with diabetes achieve better glycemic control and less medication by lowering excess fatty tissue and improving metabolic health.

HYPERTENSION (HIGH BLOOD PRESSURE):

♡ Losing weight following Dr. Nowzaradan's eating plan can lower blood pressure since excess body weight is a risk factor for hypertension.

♡ The eating plan can assist people with hypertension in achieving lower blood pressure readings and lowering their risk of heart disease and stroke by improving cardiovascular health and lessening the burden on the heart and blood vessels.

HYPERLIPIDEMIA (HIGH CHOLESTEROL):

♡ Dyslipidemia, which includes elevated levels of triglycerides and LDL cholesterol, is linked to obesity and poor dietary practices. To optimize lipid profiles, Dr. Nowzaradan's diet plan emphasizes eating more nutrient-dense, whole foods and reducing high-calorie, high-fat items.

♡ The eating plan can encourage weight loss and metabolic health, helping people achieve healthier cholesterol levels and lower their risk of atherosclerosis and cardiovascular disease.

NONALCOHOLIC FATTY LIVER DISEASE (NAFLD):

♡ People who have metabolic syndrome and obesity are more likely to have nonalcoholic fatty liver disease. Dr. Nowzaradan's diet plan can help reduce liver fat and enhance liver function if you lose weight quickly.

♡ The eating plan can assist people with nonalcoholic fatty liver disease (NAFLD) improve their liver enzyme levels and lower their risk of liver inflammation and fibrosis by encouraging a reduction in belly fat and enhancing metabolic health.

SLEEP APNEA:

♡ Obesity is a significant risk factor for sleep apnea, a disorder that causes breathing pauses during sleep. Following Dr. Nowzaradan's diet plan, weight loss can help lessen sleep apnea symptoms by reducing neck circumference and enhancing airway patency.

♡ The eating plan can enhance overall sleep patterns and daily functioning by promoting better sleep quality and minimizing the degree of sleep apnea.

JOINT DISCOMFORT AND OSTEOARTHRITIS:

♡ Being overweight puts more strain on the joints, which can cause osteoarthritis and joint discomfort. Dr. Nowzaradan's eating plan can help patients lose weight and enhance their mobility and pain management by reducing inflammation and applying joint pressure.

♡ The eating plan can assist people with joint pain and osteoarthritis to achieve better functional outcomes and lessen their need for pain medications by encouraging weight loss and maintaining a healthy body weight.

TRICKS AND TIPS FOR NOT STOPPING FOLLOWING IT

It takes commitment, tenacity, and a proactive attitude to conquer obstacles to stick to Dr. Nowzaradan's diet plan. The following are some pointers and advice to help you stick to the diet plan and not give up:

SET REALISTIC GOALS:

Set realistic short—and long-term goals for your weight loss journey. Break down more ambitious goals into smaller, more doable benchmarks to keep yourself motivated and progress-focused.

STAY CONSISTENT:
Adhere to the tenets of Dr. Nowzaradan's nutrition plan, even on weekends and special occasions. Making exceptions or overindulging in harmful meals might impede your progress, so refrain from doing so.

MAKE A MEAL PLAN:
Plan your meals and snacks to avoid eating unhealthy or impulsive foods. Prepare meals in bulk to ensure that wholesome meals are accessible throughout the week.

PRACTICE PORTION CONTROL:
To prevent overindulging, precisely measure and portion your food. To manage portion sizes and mislead your brain into thinking that you are content with less food, use smaller bowls, plates, and utensils.

KEEP HEALTHY SNACKS HANDY:
Stock up on nutritious snacks like fruits, veggies, Greek yogurt, almonds, and seeds that complement Dr. Nowzaradan's diet plan. Keep these snacks close at hand to quell hunger between meals and avoid cravings for harmful foods.

STAY HYDRATED:
Sip lots of water throughout the day to prevent hunger pangs and stay hydrated. Drink at least eight to ten glasses of water daily, and avoid sugar-filled drinks and caffeine overindulgence.

FIND HEALTHY ALTERNATIVES:
Look for healthier substitutes for your favorite meals to satiate cravings without going off your diet. For instance, replace high-calorie snacks with lower-calorie alternatives like hummus-topped veggie sticks or air-popped popcorn.

PRACTICE MINDFUL EATING:
Pay attention to your eating patterns and your body's signals of hunger and fullness. To improve enjoyment and avoid overindulging, take your time, enjoy every bite, and pay attention to the flavors and textures of your food.

SEEK SUPPORT:
♡ Encircle yourself with friends, family, or a weight loss support group that can motivate, hold you accountable, and encourage you.
♡ Join online forums or support groups to interact with people following Dr. Nowzaradan's eating plan and exchange experiences, advice, and success stories.

STAY POSITIVE AND PERSISTENT:
Pay attention to your steps and acknowledge your accomplishments along the road. Remind yourself of the reasons you began your weight loss journey and maintain your optimistic attitude in the face of obstacles or disappointments.

Remember that consistency and perseverance are essential for long-term success, and be resilient and persistent in the face of adversity.

HOW TO FOLLOW THE DIET EVEN IF YOU HANG OUT WITH FRIENDS AND FAMILY OFTEN

Sticking to Dr. Nowzaradan's food plan while interacting with friends and family can be difficult. Still, it is possible to do so without feeling deprived if you prepare ahead and communicate well. The following techniques will assist you in navigating social events while following the diet:

MAKE A PLAN:
Examine the menu or determine the available meal options before attending social gatherings. Please recommend any eateries or locations that provide healthier options per Dr. Nowzaradan's diet regimen.

EXPRESS YOUR NEEDS:
Let your loved ones know what foods you want to eat and how you want to lose weight. Ensure they understand any rules or limitations you adhere to, and solicit their assistance in choosing healthier options.

BRING YOUR FOOD:
If you're having dinner at someone's house or attending a potluck-style event, consider bringing one or two dishes that fit into Dr. Nowzaradan's diet. This guarantees that you can enjoy the meal without sacrificing your progress and that you have access to better selections.

PUT AN EMPHASIS ON PROTEIN AND VEGETABLES:
At get-togethers, prefer foods high in protein, such as fish, grilled chicken, lean meats, and non-starchy veggies. Piling these nutrient-dense foods onto your plate will sate your hunger and help you reach your weight loss objectives.

EXERCISE PORTION CONTROL:
Pay attention to serving sizes and refrain from overindulging, particularly when tempted by meals high in calories or fat. Use smaller plates and utensils to regulate portion sizes and pace yourself during the meal.

LIMIT ALCOHOL CONSUMPTION:
Due to their high-calorie content, alcoholic drinks may interfere with your attempts to lose weight. If you drink, choose lower-calorie options like herbal tea, light beer, or sparkling water with lemon or lime.

CHOOSE YOUR TREATS WISELY:
If desserts or other sweets are provided, choose smaller servings or healthier choices if better options are available. Think about splitting a dessert with someone else to fulfill your sweet taste without going overboard.

REMAIN HYDRATED:
Sip lots of water during the social event to help manage hunger and stay hydrated. Avoid sugar-filled beverages and excessive alcohol intake, as these can add needless calories.

PUT THE SOCIALIZATION FRONT AND CENTER:
Make meaningful conversations with friends and family the main attraction during get-togethers instead of the food. To spend quality time together, have conversations, participate in activities, or recommend non-food-related events.

ENGAGE IN MINDFUL EATING:
Be aware of your eating patterns and your body's signals of hunger and fullness. To avoid overeating and encourage contentment, take your time eating, enjoy every meal, and pay attention to your body's cues.

By practicing these techniques and making thoughtful decisions, you can follow Dr. Nowzaradan's food plan and still enjoy social interactions with friends and family. Remember that balance and consistency are essential, and don't be scared to speak up in social situations for your health and well-being.

THE MINDSET FOR SUCCESS

Dr. Nowzaradan's diet plan demands more than just following meal instructions to be successful; it also calls for developing a resilient and optimistic mindset. This chapter will examine the mental techniques and mindsets that support sustained success in improving health and weight loss.

WHY IT'S IMPORTANT TO SHIFT YOUR MINDSET?
Adopting a positive outlook is essential for successful weight loss that lasts. It lays the groundwork for forming wholesome routines, conquering obstacles, and retaining motivation.

KEEP YOUR GOAL IN MIND AT ALL TIMES
As you overcome obstacles and disappointments, always remember your ultimate objective. Let your image of the health, energy, and self-assurance you will acquire from reaching your weight loss objectives inspire you to keep going.

CURRENTLY IMAGINE THAT YOU ARE THE PERSON YOU WISH TO BE.
Develop a confident and self-assured outlook. Imagine yourself as the fit, energetic person you want to be, and have faith in your capacity to achieve your goals by working hard and persistently toward your goals.

EMBRACE CHANGES SINCE THEY'RE BENEFICIAL
Accept change as a necessary and constructive aspect of your path. Acknowledge that although changing your lifestyle and forming healthy habits may force you to venture outside of your comfort zone, each stride forward moves you one step closer to your objectives and a higher standard of living.

MODIFY A SINGLE HABIT AT A TIME
Instead of completely remodeling your lifestyle at once, concentrate on making little, sustainable improvements over time. Initially, focus on changing one particular habit or behavior, like eating better or getting more exercise, and then progressively build on your accomplishments over time.

DR. NOWZARADAN'S BEGINNER'S DIET PLAN
For novices, it's essential to start small. Learn about Dr. Nowzaradan's nutrition plan principles first, then progressively adopt them into your everyday routine. Remain dedicated to your objectives and acknowledge little accomplishments along the route.

STRATEGIES FOR CONQUERING SELF-DOUBT
Concentrate on your accomplishments and past qualities to counteract negative self-talk and self-doubt. Remind yourself of your past achievements and the challenges you overcame. Ascend to a group of people who will support and inspire you.

THE INFLUENCE OF HAPPINESS AND GRATITUDE
Every day, cultivate positivity and thankfulness. Maintain a thankfulness diary where you write down all the things, no matter how tiny, for which you are grateful. Maintain a positive attitude by concentrating on the things you can control and looking for the bright side of difficult circumstances.

OVERCOMING ADVERSITY AND ADAPTABILITY
Consider failures as teaching moments rather than as mistakes. Consider what caused the setback, pinpoint areas that need work, and modify your strategy accordingly. Develop resilience by overcoming setbacks with greater vigor and resolve to accomplish your objectives.

THE PATH TO SELF-REVELATION
Accept the process of self-improvement and self-discovery that comes with starting a weight loss quest. Make the most of obstacles and failures to gain new insights into your personality, assets, and potential.

If you want to follow Dr. Nowzaradan's diet plan for the long run, you must cultivate a successful attitude. By adopting a positive outlook, setting reasonable objectives, and accepting change, you may overcome challenges, maintain motivation, and eventually reach your desired level of health and wellness. Recall that everything is achievable if you put in the effort and believe you can accomplish your goals. Success starts with this belief.

WHY CHANGING MINDSET IS CRITICAL

For various reasons, changing one's perspective is essential for following Dr. Nowzaradan's diet plan.

MOTIVATION AND DETERMINATION:
A positive outlook gives you the drive and resolve to stick with your weight loss plans despite difficulties and disappointments.

ADOPTING HEALTHY HABITS:
Mindset modification entails adjusting your attitudes and convictions toward nutrition, physical activity, and self-care. A wellness-oriented mindset increases your likelihood of implementing healthy behaviors like self-care, mindful eating, and regular exercise.

OVERCOMING SELF-LIMITING BELIEFS:
Many people struggle with self-limiting ideas that get in the way of their attempts to lose weight, including "I'll never be able to lose weight" or "I always fail at diets." One must confront these unfavorable ideas and replace them with uplifting and positive views to change one's thinking.

BUILDING CONFIDENCE AND SELF-EFFICACY:
A positive outlook increases self-efficacy and confidence, or the conviction that you can succeed. Developing an optimistic outlook that emphasizes your abilities, past accomplishments, and potential for development will help you face obstacles with more self-assurance and fortitude.

MANAGING STRESS AND EMOTIONAL EATING:
Adopting a different perspective can help you learn more effective coping mechanisms for handling stress and emotional eating. You'll discover healthy coping mechanisms by learning to recognize and deal with underlying emotions rather than resorting to food as a comfort or stress reliever.

CREATING LASTING CHANGE:
A fundamental change in thinking and lifestyle is necessary for sustainable weight loss beyond simply adhering to a diet plan. By altering your perspective, you increase your chances of forming enduring behaviors that promote your health and well-being.

Adopting a different attitude is essential to following Dr. Nowzaradan's eating plan successfully because it gives you the drive, tenacity, and confidence to succeed. A positive outlook prioritizing health and well-being will help you overcome challenges, gain self-assurance, and make long-lasting changes in your life.

NEVER LOSE SIGHT OF YOUR GOAL

Maintaining your concentration, motivation, and commitment to your weight reduction journey on Dr. Nowzaradan's eating plan requires you always to keep sight of your objective. This is the reason it's crucial:

MAINTAINS MOTIVATION:
Your goal is a source of inspiration and motivation because it reminds you of the original reason you started your weight reduction journey. Recalling your objective helps rekindle your resolve to continue your current course despite obstacles or disappointments.

GIVES YOU DIRECTION:
Having a well-defined objective offers you a feeling of purpose and direction. It supports you in setting priorities for your activities, making wise choices, and maintaining focus on your goals of improving your health and well-being.

MEASURES DEVELOPMENT:
Throughout the process, you can use your goal as a standard to gauge your success and development. By regularly documenting your accomplishments and milestones, you may celebrate your successes and maintain motivation to keep moving toward your ultimate objective.

ESTABLISHES RESPONSIBILITY:
Sharing your objective with loved ones, friends, or a support group helps establish responsibility. Knowing that others know your aim might spur you to maintain commitment and take responsibility for your activities.

ENCOURAGES RESILIENCE:
A well-defined and inspiring objective will help you become more resilient and persistent when facing difficulties. It will remind you that setbacks are only transient roadblocks on the way to achievement and inspire you to keep moving forward in the face of adversity.

PROMOTES POSITIVE HABITS:
Keeping your objective in mind motivates you to adopt constructive routines and actions to help you lose weight. Your goal is a continual reminder to prioritize self-care and well-being, whether eating better, exercising frequently, or engaging in mindfulness exercises.

Maintaining your motivation, attention, and commitment to your weight reduction journey on Dr. Nowzaradan's diet plan depends on always keeping your goal in sight. By keeping your goal at the forefront of your thoughts, you can stay motivated, track your progress, establish responsibility, build resilience, and ultimately achieve your health and wellness objectives.

ALREADY SEE YOURSELF AS THE PERSON YOU WANT TO BE

A significant mental adjustment that can speed up your success on Dr. Nowzaradan's eating plan is to already envision yourself as the person you want to be. This is why it's crucial:

POSITIVE SELF-IMAGE:
You are creating a picture of the person you want to help you believe in and feel good about yourself. When you believe in yourself, you're more likely to exhibit health, fitness, and vibrancy in your choices and behaviors.

INSPIRATION AND MOTIVATION:
Seeing yourself in the future might inspire and motivate you. It helps you see your objectives clearly and reminds you of the advantages and satisfaction of reaching your weight loss objectives.

ALIGNMENT WITH GOALS:
When you see yourself as the person you wish to be, your feelings, ideas, and behaviors will align with your objectives. This reaffirms your resolve to make decisions that promote your health and well-being in the face of temptation or misfortune.

OVERCOMING LIMITING BELIEFS:
Seeing oneself as your ideal self can help you overcome self-doubt and limiting beliefs. Positive affirmations and empowering beliefs about your potential for success are used to counter negative thinking.

CREATING A BLUEPRINT FOR SUCCESS:
When you perceive yourself that way, you're more likely to adopt habits and behaviors that support your desired self-image. This develops a success blueprint that directs your choices and actions toward reaching your intended results.

ENHANCING SELF-CONFIDENCE:
Having a positive self-image helps you feel more assured and confident. It strengthens your potential for growth and transformation and gives you confidence that you can accomplish your objectives.

Conclusively, envisioning yourself as the person you desire to be is a potent mental adjustment that synchronizes your ideas, emotions, and behaviors with your objective of losing weight. Visualizing your future self can help you become more motivated, break through limiting beliefs, make a plan for success, and feel more confident as you travel toward improved health and well-being.

ACCEPT CHANGES BECAUSE THEY ARE POSITIVE

Achieving success on your weight reduction journey and adhering to Dr. Nowzaradan's diet plan requires you to embrace changes since they are positive. This is the reason it's crucial:

EMBRACING GROWTH:
Personal development and transformation are encouraged when constructive changes are accepted. Realizing the advantages of embracing healthy routines and behaviors allows you to be more receptive to opportunities and experiences that enhance your general well-being.

IMPROVING ADAPTABILITY:
Accepting constructive changes encourages resilience and adaptability in the face of difficulties. Knowing that each shift moves you closer to your goals helps you deal with changes and setbacks more easily.

DEVELOPING A GROWTH MINDSET:
A growth mindset is necessary for learning and development and is cultivated through accepting good changes. You perceive obstacles as chances for personal development and advancement rather than impassable hurdles.

ENHANCING SELF-EFFICACY:
Faith in your ability to succeed is enhanced when you embrace positive changes. Acknowledging the beneficial effects of your decisions and actions can help you gain confidence in reaching your weight loss objectives.

BUILDING MOMENTUM:
Progress is fueled by momentum, created when constructive changes are accepted. As you make significant changes one after the other, your weight reduction journey gains momentum, strengthening your dedication to better living.

BOOSTING CONTENTMENT:
Accepting constructive changes promotes more fulfillment and contentment. When you see the results of your hard work, you feel pride and satisfaction, which inspires you to keep improving your life.

To sum up, adopting Dr. Nowzaradan's diet plan and succeeding on your weight loss journey require you to accept changes because they are favorable. You may overcome challenges, gain confidence, and bring about long-lasting change by realizing the advantages of adopting better habits and behaviors, encouraging flexibility and resilience, and developing a growth mindset.

CHANGE ONE HABIT AT A TIME

A calculated strategy that can result in long-term success on Dr. Nowzaradan's diet plan is to modify one habit at a time. This is the reason it's crucial:

CLARITY AND FOCUS:
Breaking a habit one at a time enables you to concentrate your attention and energy on a particular activity, which makes it simpler to carry out and maintain in the long run. By keeping things focused, you may identify your priorities clearly and avoid becoming overwhelmed.

INCREMENTAL PROGRESS:
You can approach your weight loss objectives incrementally by focusing on one behavior at a time. Over time, your little adjustments can significantly impact your general health and well-being.

CREATING ROUTINES:
Modifying one behavior at a time can help you create new routines and habits to reduce your weight. Healthy habits become instinctive and embedded when you adopt them into your daily routine, making them more straightforward to stick with over time.

GAINING CONFIDENCE:
Successfully changing just one behavior gives you a sense of achievement and increases your confidence in your capacity to make healthy adjustments. This self-assurance might spur you to break other destructive behaviors and keep moving closer to your objectives.

FINDING SUCCESSFUL STRATEGIES:
You can test several methods and techniques for changing your behavior by concentrating on one habit at a time. Based on your experiences and results, you may determine what works best for you and improve your strategy.

PREVENTING OVERWHELM:
Attempting to modify too many habits at once can result in burnout and overwhelm. By prioritizing one habit at a time, you can prevent feeling overwhelmed and keep your sense of control and momentum while losing weight.

Modifying a single habit at a time is a realistic and successful strategy for adhering to Dr. Nowzaradan's diet plan. By concentrating your efforts, making small but steady improvements, and gaining confidence, you can create healthy habits that promote your long-term health and well-being.

DR. NOWZARADAN'S DIET PLAN FOR BEGINNERS

Welcome to Dr. Nowzaradan's Diet Plan for Beginners! If you're reading this, you've taken the first step towards improving your health and embarking on a transformative journey towards sustainable weight loss. Dr. Nowzaradan, a renowned bariatric surgeon and weight loss specialist, has helped countless individuals achieve their weight loss goals and reclaim their lives through his proven diet plan.

BREAKFAST RECIPES

VEGGIE OMELETTE

COOKING TIME: 15 MINUTES, SERVING: 1 SERVING

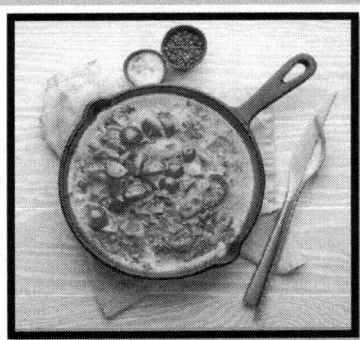

This veggie omelet is packed with fresh vegetables, providing a nutrient-rich, low-calorie breakfast option that is satisfying and healthy.

INGREDIENTS:
- Two egg whites
- One whole egg
- 1/4 cup diced bell peppers
- 1/4 cup diced onions
- 1/4 cup diced tomatoes
- 1/4 cup spinach
- Salt and pepper to taste
- Cooking spray or 1 tsp olive oil

STEP-BY-STEP INSTRUCTIONS:
1. In a bowl, whisk together the whole egg and the egg whites. Season with salt and pepper.
2. Grease a non-stick skillet with cooking spray or olive oil and heat it over medium heat.
3. Add the chopped bell peppers, onions, and tomatoes to the skillet and sauté until the vegetables are soft, three to four minutes.
4. Cook the spinach for another one to two minutes or until it wilts.
5. Over the veggies in the skillet, pour the egg mixture.
6. Allow the raw egg to flow below by gently raising the sides with a spatula and cooking for 3–4 minutes.
7. After the eggs are ready, slide the omelet onto a platter by folding it in half.

BENEFITS:
This omelet is packed with fiber and protein, making a filling and healthy breakfast.

NUTRITION PLAN: PER SERVING
Calories: 150, Protein: 18g, Carbohydrates: 6g, Fat: 6g,

GREEK YOGURT PARFAIT

COOKING TIME: 5 MINUTES, SERVING: 1 SERVING

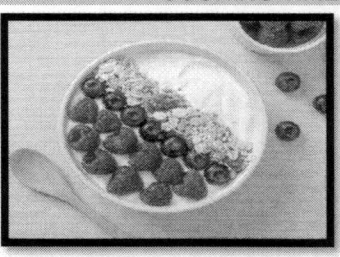

For a protein-packed breakfast, a refreshing parfait layered with Greek yogurt, fresh berries, and a sprinkle of nuts.

INGREDIENTS:
- 1 cup Greek yogurt (non-fat)
- 1/2 cup fresh berries (strawberries, blueberries, or raspberries)
- 2 tbsp chopped nuts (almonds, walnuts, or pecans)

STEP-BY-STEP INSTRUCTIONS:
1. Place one-third cup of Greek yogurt in a glass or bowl.
2. Half of the fresh berries should be layered over the yogurt.
3. Add one and a third cups more Greek yogurt.
4. Incorporate the leftover berries.
5. Place the last 1/3 cup of Greek yogurt on top.
6. Add some chopped nuts on the top.

BENEFITS:
Packed with protein and antioxidants, this parfait is a tasty and nutritious way to start the day.

NUTRITION PLAN: PER SERVING
Calories: 200, Protein: 20g, Carbohydrates: 20g, Fat: 6g

AVOCADO TOAST

COOKING TIME: 5 MINUTES, SERVING: 1 SERVING

A simple yet nutritious toast topped with mashed avocado and a drizzle of olive oil.

INGREDIENTS:
- One slice whole grain bread
- 1/2 ripe avocado
- 1 tsp olive oil
- Salt and pepper to taste

STEP-BY-STEP INSTRUCTIONS:
1. Toast the whole grain bread slice.
2. Mash the avocado in a small bowl while the bread is toasting.
3. Toast the bread and then spread the mashed avocado on it.
4. Add a drizzle of olive oil and taste-test salt and pepper for seasoning.

BENEFITS:
Avocado toast is a satisfying and speedy meal with fiber and good fats.

NUTRITION PLAN: PER SERVING
Calories: 250, Protein: 5g, Carbohydrates: 24g, Fat: 16g

PROTEIN PANCAKES

COOKING TIME: 15 MINUTES, SERVING: 2 SERVINGS

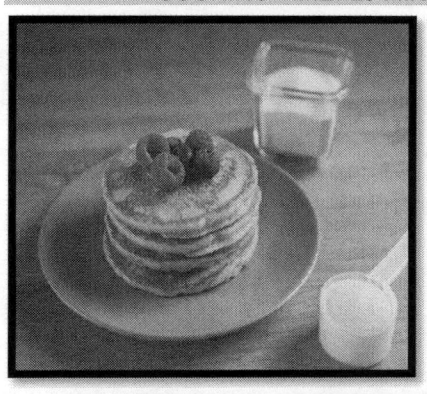

These protein pancakes are made with whole grain flour and protein powder, offering a filling and satisfying morning meal.

INGREDIENTS:
- 1/2 cup whole grain flour
- One scoop of protein powder (vanilla or plain)
- 1/2 tsp baking powder
- 1/2 cup almond milk (unsweetened)
- One egg
- 1 tsp vanilla extract
- Cooking spray or 1 tsp coconut oil

STEP-BY-STEP INSTRUCTIONS:
1. Combine the flour, baking powder, and protein powder in a bowl.
2. Whisk the egg, vanilla essence, and almond milk in a separate basin.
3. Mix the dry ingredients into the wet mixture, stirring just until incorporated.
4. Coat a non-stick skillet with coconut oil or cooking spray and heat it over medium heat.
5. For each pancake, add 1/4 cup of batter to the skillet.
6. Cook for 2 to 3 minutes on each side until bubbles appear on the surface, then turn and continue cooking until golden brown.
7. Garnish the dish with sliced strawberries and a dollop of Greek yogurt if preferred.

BENEFITS:
Packed with fiber and protein, these pancakes keep you full and focused all morning.

NUTRITION PLAN: PER SERVING
Calories: 200, Protein: 20g, Carbohydrates: 20g, Fat: 5g

Breakfast Burrito

COOKING TIME: 10 MINUTES, SERVING: 1 SERVING

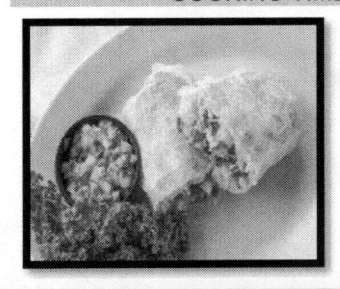

A hearty breakfast burrito filled with scrambled eggs, black beans, and salsa for a portable breakfast option.

INGREDIENTS:
- One whole-grain tortilla
- Two eggs scrambled
- 1/4 cup black beans, rinsed and drained
- 2 tbsp salsa
- 1/4 cup shredded low-fat cheese (optional)
- Cooking spray or 1 tsp olive oil

STEP-BY-STEP INSTRUCTIONS:
1. In a non-stick skillet, scramble the eggs using cooking spray or olive oil.
2. Use a skillet or a microwave to reheat the tortilla.
3. Spread the tortilla and top with the black beans, salsa, cheese (if using), and scrambled eggs.

4. Fold the tortilla's edges and roll it up to create a burrito.

BENEFITS:
Packed with fiber and protein, this breakfast burrito provides a satisfying and well-rounded meal to start the day.

NUTRITION PLAN: PER SERVING
Calories: 300, Protein: 20g, Carbohydrates: 30g, Fat: 10g

OVERNIGHT OATS

COOKING TIME: 5 MINUTES + OVERNIGHT SOAKING, SERVING: 1 SERVING

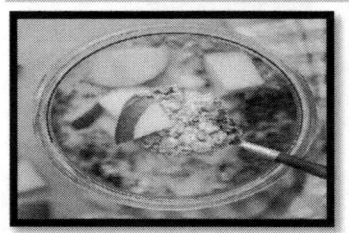

Soak rolled oats in almond milk and top with sliced fruit and cinnamon for a quick and easy breakfast.

INGREDIENTS:
- 1/2 cup rolled oats
- 1/2 cup almond milk (unsweetened)
- 1/2 apple, diced
- 1/4 tsp cinnamon
- 1 tsp honey (optional)

STEP-BY-STEP INSTRUCTIONS:
1. Combine the rolled oats and almond milk in a mixing bowl or jar.
2. Stir in the diced apples and cinnamon to mix.
3. Cover and chill overnight.
4. In the morning, mix the oats and, if desired, drizzle with honey.

BENEFITS:
Overnight oats are high in fiber and simple to cook, making them an excellent breakfast option.

NUTRITION PLAN: PER SERVING
Calories: 250, Protein: 6g, Carbohydrates: 45g, Fat: 5g

SMOOTHIE BOWL

COOKING TIME: 5 MINUTES, SERVING: 1 SERVING

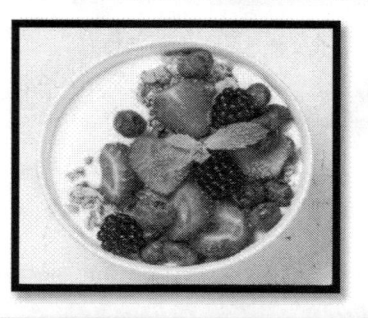

Blend frozen fruit, Greek yogurt, and spinach to make a nutrient-dense smoothie bowl topped with granola and almonds.

INGREDIENTS:
- 1 cup frozen mixed berries
- 1/2 cup Greek yogurt (non-fat)
- 1/2 cup spinach
- 1/2 banana
- 1/4 cup granola
- 2 tbsp chopped nuts

STEP-BY-STEP INSTRUCTIONS:
1. Blend the frozen berries, banana, Greek yogurt, and spinach.
2. Blend until thick and smooth.
3. Transfer into a bowl and garnish with chopped nuts and granola.

BENEFITS:

Packed with protein and antioxidants, this smoothie bowl is a tasty and nutritious way to start the day.

NUTRITION PLAN: PER SERVING
Calories: 300, Protein: 15g, Carbohydrates: 50g, Fat: 10g

CHIA SEED PUDDING

COOKING TIME: 5 MINUTES + OVERNIGHT SOAKING, SERVING: 1 SERVING

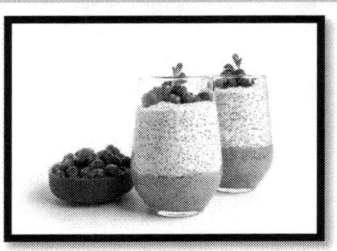

Blend almond milk and chia seeds, then add a little honey to taste. This makes a filling and healthy breakfast pudding.

INGREDIENTS:
- 3 tbsp chia seeds
- 1 cup almond milk (unsweetened)
- 1 tsp honey
- 1/4 cup fresh berries

STEP-BY-STEP INSTRUCTIONS:
1. Mix the almond milk, honey, and chia seeds in a basin or container.
2. Make sure the chia seeds are dispersed evenly by stirring it evenly dispersed by stirring them well.
3. Stir the pudding and add fresh berries on top in the morning.

BENEFITS:
Rich in omega-3 fatty acids and fiber, chia seed pudding is a wholesome and straightforward breakfast option.

NUTRITION PLAN: PER SERVING
Calories: 200, Protein: 6g, Carbohydrates: 25g, Fat: 10g

LUNCH RECIPES

GRILLED CHICKEN SALAD

COOKING TIME: 20 MINUTES, SERVING: 1 SERVING

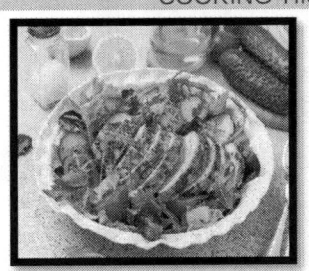

Grilled chicken breast, mixed greens, cucumbers, cherry tomatoes, and balsamic vinaigrette come together in this delightful salad.

INGREDIENTS:
- 1 grilled chicken breast
- 2 cups mixed greens
- 1/2 cup cherry tomatoes, halved
- 1/2 cucumber, sliced
- 2 tbsp balsamic vinaigrette

STEP-BY-STEP INSTRUCTIONS:
1. Grill 5 to 7 minutes on each side or until the chicken breast is cooked. After letting it rest, cut it.
2. Mix the cucumber, cherry tomatoes, and greens in a big bowl.
3. Place the grilled chicken slices on top of the salad.
4. Over the salad, drizzle with the balsamic vinaigrette and toss to mix.

BENEFITS:
This salad is a healthy and energizing lunch choice because it is high in protein and low in calories.

NUTRITION PLAN: PER SERVING
Calories: 250, Protein: 30g, Carbohydrates: 10g, Fat: 10g

QUINOA SALAD

COOKING TIME: 20 MINUTES, SERVING: 2 SERVINGS

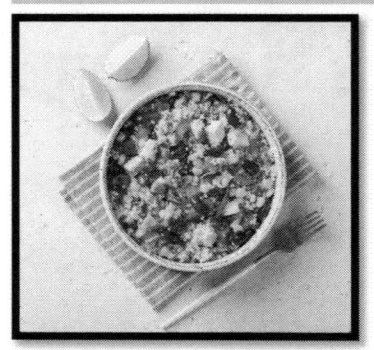

Diced veggies, chickpeas, and a dab of lemon juice are combined to create this protein- and fiber-rich quinoa salad.

INGREDIENTS:
- 1 cup cooked quinoa
- 1/2 cup diced bell peppers
- 1/2 cup diced cucumber
- 1/2 cup cherry tomatoes, halved
- 1/2 cup chickpeas, rinsed and drained
- Juice of 1 lemon
- 1 tbsp olive oil
- Salt and pepper to taste

STEP-BY-STEP INSTRUCTIONS:
1. After cooking the quinoa as directed on the package, allow it to cool.
2. The cooked quinoa, bell peppers, cucumber, cherry tomatoes, and chickpeas should all be combined in a big bowl.
3. Olive oil and lemon juice should be drizzled on.
4. Add salt and pepper to taste, then toss to mix.

BENEFITS:
Packed with fiber and protein, this quinoa salad is a hearty and nourishing lunch option.

NUTRITION PLAN: PER SERVING
Calories: 300, Protein: 10g, Carbohydrates: 40g, Fat: 10g

TURKEY LETTUCE WRAPS

COOKING TIME: 15 MINUTES, SERVING: 2 SERVINGS

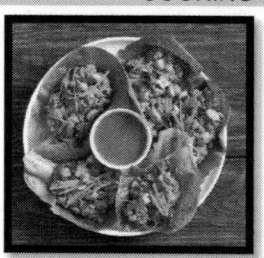

Lettuce leaves are stuffed with lean turkey breast, sliced avocado, and shredded carrots in these low-carb wraps.

INGREDIENTS:
- Four large lettuce leaves
- 8 oz lean turkey breast, sliced
- One avocado, sliced
- 1/2 cup shredded carrots
- 1 tbsp low-sodium soy sauce (optional)

STEP-BY-STEP INSTRUCTIONS:
1. On a dish, arrange the lettuce leaves.
2. Arrange sliced turkey breast, avocado, and shredded carrots on each leaf.
3. If desired, drizzle with soy sauce.
4. To make lettuce wraps, roll the leaves around the fillings.

BENEFITS:
These lettuce wraps are a filling and healthful lunch choice because they are high in protein and low in carbs.

NUTRITION PLAN: PER SERVING
Calories: 250, Protein: 20g, Carbohydrates: 15g, Fat: 15g

VEGGIE STIR-FRY

COOKING TIME: 20 MINUTES, SERVING: 2 SERVINGS

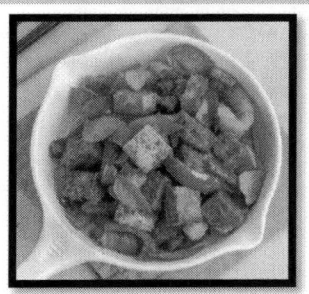

A bright and tasty stir-fry cooked with tofu and a mix of vegetables.

INGREDIENTS:
- 1 tbsp olive oil
- 1 cup broccoli florets
- One red bell pepper, sliced
- One carrot, julienned
- 1 cup snap peas
- 1/2 block firm tofu, cubed
- 2 tbsp low-sodium soy sauce

STEP-BY-STEP INSTRUCTIONS:
1. In a big skillet, warm the olive oil over medium-high heat.
2. Add the carrot, snap peas, bell pepper, and broccoli. Stir-fry for 5 to 7 minutes or until crisp-tender.
3. After adding the soy sauce and cubed tofu, simmer for three to four minutes or until thoroughly heated.

BENEFITS:
Packed with protein and fiber, this colorful and healthy veggie stir-fry is a great lunch.

NUTRITION PLAN: PER SERVING
Calories: 300, Protein: 15g, Carbohydrates: 25g, Fat: 15g

TUNA SALAD

COOKING TIME: 10 MINUTES, SERVING: 1 SERVING

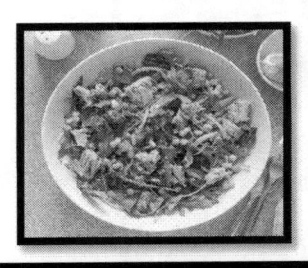

This creamy, protein-rich tuna salad combines Greek yogurt, sliced celery, mustard, and canned tuna.

INGREDIENTS:
- One can of tuna in water, drained
- 2 tbsp Greek yogurt (non-fat)
- One celery stalk, diced
- 1 tsp mustard
- Salt and pepper to taste

STEP-BY-STEP INSTRUCTIONS:
1. Combine the tuna, Greek yogurt, mustard, and diced celery in a bowl.
2. To taste, add salt and pepper for seasoning.
3. Serve with whole grain crackers or over a bed of lettuce.

BENEFITS:

This tuna salad is a filling and healthful lunch choice because it is high in protein and low in fat.

NUTRITION PLAN: PER SERVING
Calories: 200, Protein: 30g, Carbohydrates: 5g, Fat: 5g

LENTIL SOUP

COOKING TIME: 30 MINUTES, SERVING: 4 SERVINGS

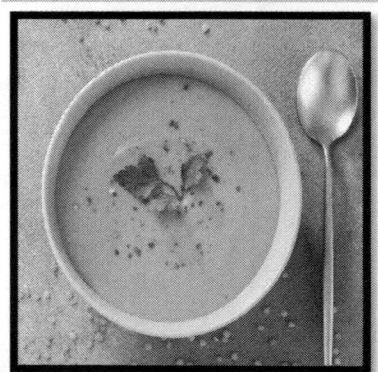

This lentil soup is filling and substantial and is made by cooking lentils with veggies and spices.

INGREDIENTS:
- 1 cup lentils, rinsed
- One onion, diced
- Two carrots diced
- Two celery stalks, diced
- Three cloves garlic, minced
- One can of diced tomatoes (14.5 oz)
- 4 cups vegetable broth
- 1 tsp cumin
- 1 tsp paprika
- Salt and pepper to taste

STEP-BY-STEP INSTRUCTIONS:
1. Add the onion, carrots, and celery to a large pot and sauté over medium heat until softened, about 5 minutes.
2. After adding the garlic, heat it for one more minute.
3. Add the paprika, cumin, diced tomatoes, vegetable broth, and lentils and stir.
4. Once the lentils are soft, boil, lower the heat, and simmer for 20 minutes.
5. Before serving, add salt and pepper to taste.

BENEFITS:
Lentil soup is a hearty and nourishing lunch choice high in protein and fiber.

NUTRITION PLAN: PER SERVING
Calories: 250, Protein: 15g, Carbohydrates: 40g, Fat: 2g

QUINOA BOWL

COOKING TIME: 30 MINUTES, SERVING: 2 SERVINGS

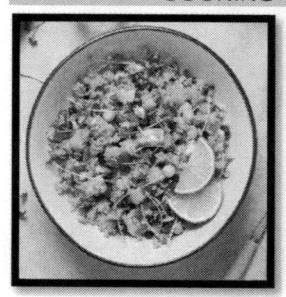

Cooked quinoa, roasted veggies, and grilled shrimp combine to make a nutritious and substantial quinoa bowl.

INGREDIENTS:
- 1 cup cooked quinoa
- 1 cup roasted vegetables (bell peppers, zucchini, cherry tomatoes)
- 8 oz shrimp, peeled and deveined
- 1 tbsp olive oil
- Juice of 1 lemon
- Salt and pepper to taste

STEP-BY-STEP INSTRUCTIONS:
1. After cooking the quinoa as directed on the package, allow it to cool.

2. Toss the vegetables with salt, pepper, and olive oil and roast for 20 minutes at 400°F.
3. Grill the shrimp on each side for two to three minutes or until done.
4. The quinoa, roasted veggies, and grilled shrimp should all be combined in a bowl.
5. Pour in some lemon juice, then toss to mix.

BENEFITS:
Packed with fiber and protein, this quinoa dish makes a healthy, well-balanced meal.

NUTRITION PLAN: PER SERVING
Calories: 350, Protein: 25g, Carbohydrates: 45g, Fat: 10g

STUFFED BELL PEPPERS

COOKING TIME: 40 MINUTES, SERVING: 4 SERVINGS

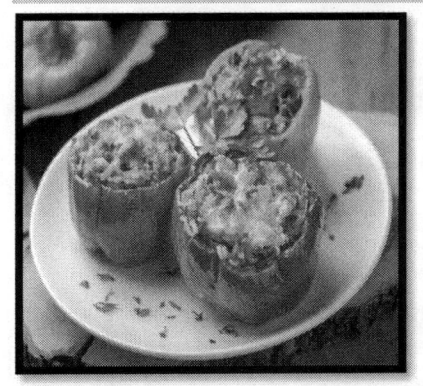

Bell peppers are portable and packed with healthy ingredients such as diced veggies, quinoa, and minced turkey.

INGREDIENTS:
- Four bell pepper tops were cut off, and the seeds were removed
- 1/2 lb ground turkey
- 1 cup cooked quinoa
- 1/2 cup diced tomatoes
- 1/2 onion, diced
- 1 cup spinach, chopped
- 1 tsp olive oil
- Salt and pepper to taste

STEP-BY-STEP INSTRUCTIONS:
1. Turn the oven on to 375°F.
2. Heat the olive oil in a pan over medium heat. Add the onion and simmer for about 5 minutes or until softened.
3. Using a spoon, break up the ground turkey as you cook it until it turns brown.
4. Add the spinach, cooked quinoa, and diced tomatoes and stir. Cook until wilted, about 3 minutes.
5. To taste, add salt and pepper for seasoning.
6. Stuff the turkey-quinoa mixture inside the bell peppers.
7. After placing the filled peppers in a baking tray, bake them for 20 to 25 minutes or until they become soft.

BENEFITS:
Packed with fiber and protein, these stuffed bell peppers are a filling and healthful lunch choice.

NUTRITION PLAN: PER SERVING
Calories: 300, Protein: 20g, Carbohydrates: 30g, Fat: 10g

DINNER RECIPES

BAKED SALMON

COOKING TIME: 25 MINUTES, SERVING: 2 SERVINGS

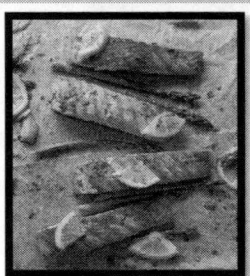

Salmon fillets make a simple and quick supper when seasoned with herbs and lemon juice and baked until soft and flaky.

INGREDIENTS:
- ☐ Two salmon fillets (about 6 oz each)
- ☐ One lemon, juiced
- ☐ 1 tsp olive oil
- ☐ 1 tsp dried dill
- ☐ Salt and pepper to taste

STEP-BY-STEP INSTRUCTIONS:
1. Turn the oven on to 375°F, or 190°C.
2. Arrange the salmon fillets on a parchment paper-lined baking pan.
3. Pour olive oil and lemon juice over the salmon.
4. Add some pepper, salt, and dill.
5. Salmon should flake easily with a fork and be cooked through after 20 minutes in the oven.

BENEFITS:
Rich in protein and omega-3 fatty acids, this dish offers vital nutrients and promotes heart health.

NUTRITION PLAN: PER SERVING
Calories: 300, Protein: 34g, Carbohydrates: 2g, Fat: 18g

TURKEY MEATBALLS

COOKING TIME: 30 MINUTES, SERVING: 4 SERVINGS

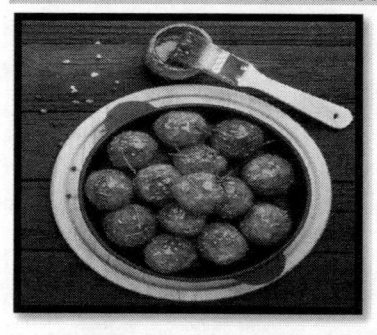

Roll ground turkey into meatballs and bake in marinara sauce for a protein-packed and flavorful dinner.

INGREDIENTS:
- ☐ 1 lb ground turkey
- ☐ 1/2 cup breadcrumbs (whole grain or gluten-free)
- ☐ One egg
- ☐ 1/4 cup grated Parmesan cheese
- ☐ 1 tsp dried Italian herbs
- ☐ 2 cups marinara sauce

STEP-BY-STEP INSTRUCTIONS:
1. Turn the oven on to 400°F or 200°C.
2. Thoroughly mix ground turkey, breadcrumbs, egg, Parmesan cheese, and Italian herbs in a basin.
3. Place mixture on a baking sheet and roll into 1-inch meatballs.
4. Meatballs should be baked for 15 to 20 minutes to ensure doneness.

5. Warm the marinara sauce in a skillet over medium heat.
6. Simmer the cooked meatballs in the sauce for five minutes.

BENEFITS:
This recipe is a high-protein, low-fat supper option thanks to the lean protein from the turkey.

NUTRITION PLAN: PER SERVING
Calories: 250, Protein: 30g, Carbohydrates: 15g, Fat: 8g

STIR-FRIED TOFU

COOKING TIME: 20 MINUTES, SERVING: 2 SERVINGS

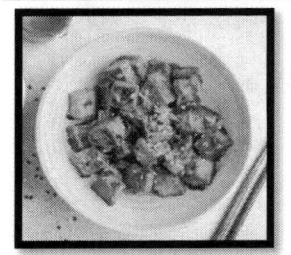

An enjoyable plant-based supper option is to stir-fry tofu with veggies and teriyaki sauce.

INGREDIENTS:
- One block of firm tofu cubed
- 1 tbsp olive oil
- One red bell pepper, sliced
- 1 cup broccoli florets
- One carrot, julienned
- 1/4 cup teriyaki sauce

STEP-BY-STEP INSTRUCTIONS:
1. Warm up the olive oil in a big skillet set over medium-high heat.
2. In around five minutes, add the tofu cubes and cook until golden brown.
3. Add the carrot, broccoli, and bell pepper to the skillet.
4. Once the veggies are soft, stir-fry them for five to seven minutes.
5. Drizzle the tofu and veggies with teriyaki sauce, ensuring everything is uniformly coated.

BENEFITS:
Packed with fiber and plant-based protein, this dish promotes healthy digestion and muscles.

NUTRITION PLAN: PER SERVING
Calories: 300, Protein: 20g, Carbohydrates: 20g, Fat: 15g

CHICKEN STIR-FRY

COOKING TIME: 20 MINUTES, SERVING: 2 SERVINGS

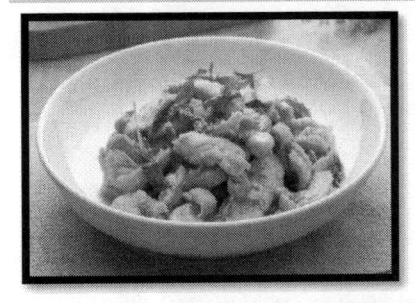

A quick and healthful stir-fry dinner can be made by sautéing chicken breast with assorted vegetables and a little soy sauce.

INGREDIENTS:
- Two chicken breasts, thinly sliced
- 1 tbsp olive oil
- 1 cup snap peas
- One red bell pepper, sliced
- One carrot, julienned
- 2 tbsp low-sodium soy sauce

STEP-BY-STEP INSTRUCTIONS:
1. Warm up the olive oil in a big skillet set over medium-high heat.

2. Cook the chicken slices for 5 to 7 minutes until they are no longer pink.
3. Add bell pepper, carrot, and snap peas to the skillet.
4. Once the veggies are soft, stir-fry them for five to seven minutes.
5. Pour in the soy sauce and mix everything.

BENEFITS:
This stir-fry is a healthy, well-balanced supper that is high in protein and low in fat.

NUTRITION PLAN: PER SERVING
Calories: 300, Protein: 35g, Carbohydrates: 10g, Fat: 12g

GRILLED VEGGIE SKEWERS

COOKING TIME: 30 MINUTES, SERVING: 4 SERVINGS

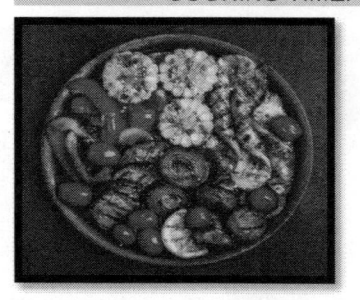

A beautiful and savory dinner can be prepared by grilling bell peppers, zucchini, mushrooms, and cherry tomatoes on skewers.

INGREDIENTS:
- Two bell peppers, cut into chunks
- Two zucchinis, sliced
- 1 cup mushrooms, halved
- 1 cup cherry tomatoes
- 2 tbsp olive oil
- Salt and pepper to taste

STEP-BY-STEP INSTRUCTIONS:
1. Grill at a medium-high temperature.
2. Cherry tomatoes, bell peppers, zucchini, and mushrooms should all be skewered.
3. Apply a thin layer of olive oil and sprinkle with salt and pepper.
4. When the vegetables are soft and beginning to caramelize, grill the skewers for 10 to 12 minutes, rotating them halfway through.

BENEFITS:
Packed with vitamins and antioxidants, these vegetable skewers promote general well-being.

NUTRITION PLAN: PER SERVING
Calories: 150, Protein: 4g, Carbohydrates: 15g, Fat: 9g

SPAGHETTI SQUASH WITH MARINARA

COOKING TIME: 45 MINUTES, SERVING: 4 SERVINGS

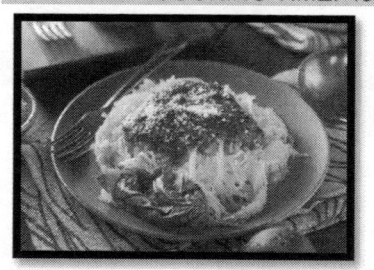

Roast spaghetti squash and top with marinara sauce and grated Parmesan cheese for a low-carb and satisfying pasta alternative.

INGREDIENTS:
- One large spaghetti squash
- 2 cups marinara sauce
- 1/4 cup grated Parmesan cheese
- 1 tbsp olive oil
- Salt and pepper to taste

STEP-BY-STEP INSTRUCTIONS:
1. Turn the oven on to 400°F or 200°C.

2. Scoop out the seeds after cutting the spaghetti squash in half lengthwise.
3. Put the sliced side on a baking sheet, drizzle with olive oil, and season with salt and pepper.
4. Roast until soft, about 40 minutes.
5. Scrape the squash strands into a bowl using a fork.
6. In a saucepan, warm the marinara sauce over medium heat.
7. Serve spaghetti squash with Parmesan cheese and marinara sauce on top.

BENEFITS:
This dish is a healthy substitute for regular pasta because it is high in fiber and low in carbs.

NUTRITION PLAN: PER SERVING
Calories: 200, Protein: 6g, Carbohydrates: 30g, Fat: 8g

CAULIFLOWER FRIED RICE

COOKING TIME: 20 MINUTES, SERVING: 4 SERVINGS

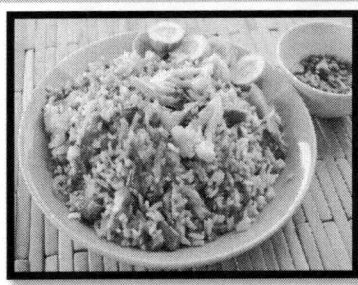

A healthier alternative to fried rice is to pulse cauliflower in a food processor and stir-fry it with vegetables, eggs, and soy sauce.

INGREDIENTS:
- One large cauliflower, riced
- 2 tbsp olive oil
- 1 cup peas and carrots (frozen or fresh)
- Two eggs, beaten
- 2 tbsp low-sodium soy sauce
- One green onion, sliced

STEP-BY-STEP INSTRUCTIONS:
1. In a food processor, pulse cauliflower until it resembles rice.
2. Warm up the olive oil in a big skillet set over medium-high heat.
3. Cook the carrots and peas for five minutes or until they are soft.
4. After pushing the veggies to one side of the skillet, add the beaten eggs and scramble until they are done.
5. Stir together the soy sauce and the riced cauliflower.
6. Cook until the cauliflower is soft, about five more minutes.
7. Add sliced green onions as a garnish.

BENEFITS:
This dish is a healthy and filling substitute for regular fried rice because it is low in calories and fiber.

NUTRITION PLAN: PER SERVING
Calories: 150, Protein: 6g, Carbohydrates: 15g, Fat: 8g

TURKEY CHILI

COOKING TIME: 45 MINUTES, SERVING: 4 SERVINGS

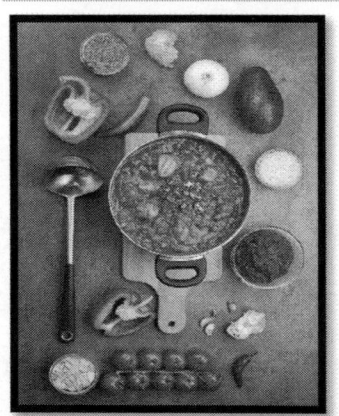

An easy and satisfying chili meal alternative is to simmer ground turkey with tomatoes, beans, and spices.

INGREDIENTS:
- 1 lb ground turkey
- One onion, diced
- One bell pepper, diced
- Two cloves garlic, minced
- One can of diced tomatoes (14.5 oz)
- One can of kidney beans (14.5 oz), rinsed and drained
- 1 tbsp chili powder
- 1 tsp cumin
- Salt and pepper to taste

STEP-BY-STEP INSTRUCTIONS:
1. Cook the ground turkey in a big pot over medium heat for 5 to 7 minutes or until browned.
2. Add the onion, bell pepper, and garlic, and simmer for about 5 minutes or until the vegetables are tender.
3. Add kidney beans, cumin, chili powder, and diced tomatoes and stir.
4. After reaching a boil, lower the heat and simmer for 30 minutes.
5. To taste, add salt and pepper for seasoning.

BENEFITS:
Packed with fiber and lean protein, this turkey chili is a hearty and nourishing dish for chilly days.

NUTRITION PLAN: PER SERVING
Calories: 250, Protein: 25g, Carbohydrates: 20g, Fat: 8g

SNACKS

CELERY STICKS WITH ALMOND BUTTER

COOKING TIME: 5 MINUTES, SERVING: 1 SERVING

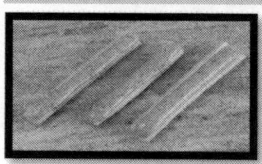

Creamy almond butter-filled celery sticks provide a crisp snack with fiber and good fats.

INGREDIENTS:
- Celery sticks
- Almond butter

STEP-BY-STEP INSTRUCTIONS:
1. Clean the celery and chop it into sticks.
2. Apply a layer of almond butter to every celery stick.
3. Present and savor!

BENEFITS:

This snack fits well with Dr. Nowzaradan's beginner's diet plan because it's easy to increase fiber consumption and boost energy.

NUTRITION PLAN: PER SERVING
Calories: 150, Protein: 5g, Carbohydrates: 10g, Fat: 10g

ALMONDS

COOKING TIME: NONE, SERVING: 1 SERVING (28 GRAMS)

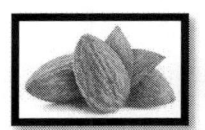

Almonds are a filling and nutritious snack packed with protein and good fats.

INGREDIENTS:
- Almonds

STEP-BY-STEP INSTRUCTIONS:
1. All you have to do is grab a handful of almonds and nibble on them quickly and conveniently.

BENEFITS:
Packed with protein, fiber, and other essential nutrients, almonds are a terrific choice for boosting satiety and giving you energy that lasts all day.

NUTRITION PLAN: PER SERVING
Calories: 160, Protein: 6g, Carbohydrates: 6g, Fat: 14g

GREEK YOGURT

COOKING TIME: NONE, SERVING: 1 SERVING (ABOUT 245 GRAMS)

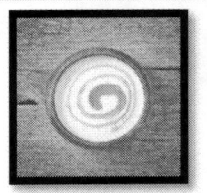

Greek yogurt is a creamy, high-protein snack that tastes great with sliced fruit and honey drizzled over it.

INGREDIENTS:
- Greek yogurt
- Honey
- Sliced fruit (such as berries or bananas)

STEP-BY-STEP INSTRUCTIONS:
- Fill a bowl with Greek yogurt.
- Pour honey on top of the yogurt.
- Add sliced fruit on top.
- Have fun!

BENEFITS:
Greek yogurt keeps you full and content while offering substantial protein, calcium, and probiotics to support digestive health and muscular strength.

NUTRITION PLAN: PER SERVING
Calories: 200, Protein: 20g, Carbohydrates: 25g, Fat: 2g

BABY CARROTS AND HUMMUS

SERVING: 10 BABY CARROTS & 2 TABLESPOONS HUMMUS

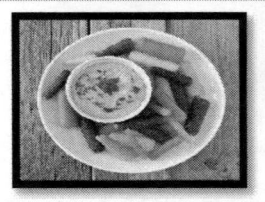

Hummus and baby carrots combine to create a crisp, filling, high-fiber, and protein snack.

INGREDIENTS:
- ☐ Baby carrots
- ☐ Hummus

STEP-BY-STEP INSTRUCTIONS:
1. Thoroughly wash the baby carrots.
2. Transfer the young carrots to a platter.
3. Accompany with hummus for dipping on the side.
4. Have fun!

BENEFITS:
This snack is nutrient-dense and satisfying because baby carrots are high in fiber and low in calories, and hummus offers plant-based protein and good fats.

NUTRITION PLAN: PER SERVING
Calories: 100, Protein: 4g, Carbohydrates: 14g, Fat: 4g

APPLE SLICES WITH PEANUT BUTTER

SERVING: 1 MEDIUM APPLE & 2 TABLESPOONS OF PEANUT BUTTER)

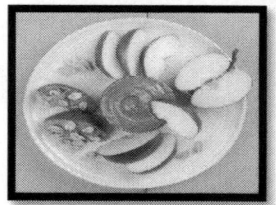

Apple slices and peanut butter combine to make a savory, sweet snack high in fiber and good fats.

INGREDIENTS:
- ☐ Apple
- ☐ Peanut butter

STEP-BY-STEP INSTRUCTIONS:
1. After washing the apple, slice it.
2. Arrange the apple slices with peanut butter on them.
3. Have fun!

BENEFITS:
This snack is satiating and nutrient-dense. Peanut butter adds protein and healthy fats, and apples are a great source of fiber and other nutrients.

NUTRITION PLAN: PER SERVING
Calories: 230, Protein: 7g, Carbohydrates: 25g, Fat: 14g

COTTAGE CHEESE WITH PINEAPPLE

SERVING: 1/2 CUP COTTAGE CHEESE & 1/2 CUP FRESH PINEAPPLE CHUNKS

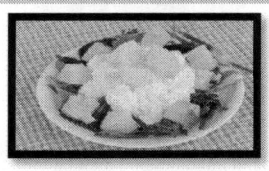

Combining cottage cheese and fresh pineapple pieces creates a tasty, protein-rich snack alternative.

INGREDIENTS:
- Cottage cheese
- Fresh pineapple chunks

STEP-BY-STEP INSTRUCTIONS:
1. Measure out the fresh pineapple pieces and cottage cheese to your preferred amount.
2. Put the pineapple pieces and cottage cheese in a bowl.
3. Gently stir everything together.
4. Have fun!

BENEFITS:
Pineapple adds natural sweetness and vitamin C, and cottage cheese is high in calcium and protein, making this snack satiating and nourishing.

NUTRITION PLAN: PER SERVING
Calories: 160, Protein: 14g, Carbohydrates: 22g, Fat: 2g

HARD-BOILED EGGS

COOKING TIME: 10 MINUTES, SERVING: 2 EGGS

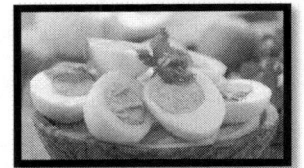

Hard-boiled eggs are a portable, high-protein snack that tastes great on the run.

INGREDIENTS:
- Eggs

STEP-BY-STEP INSTRUCTIONS:
1. Put the eggs into a pot and pour water over them.
2. Put the water on medium-high heat and bring it to a boil.
3. After the saucepan reaches a boil, put a lid on it and turn off the heat.
4. Let your eggs sit in the boiling water for nine to twelve minutes, depending on how you want them.
5. After taking the eggs out of the hot water, let them cool in a bowl of ice water.
6. After the eggs have cooled, peel them and eat!

BENEFITS:
Hard-boiled eggs are a satisfying and healthy snack option because they're a great source of protein and essential nutrients.

NUTRITION PLAN: PER SERVING
Calories: 140, Protein: 12g, Carbohydrates: 1g, Fat: 10g

EDAMAME

COOKING TIME: 5 MINUTES, SERVING: 1/2 CUP EDAMAME

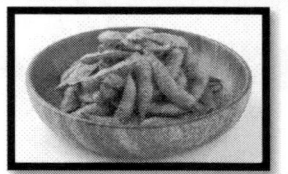

Edamame cooked in water and seasoned with sea salt is a filling and healthy snack.

INGREDIENTS:
- Edamame (frozen or fresh)
- Sea salt

STEP-BY-STEP INSTRUCTIONS:
1. When using frozen edamame, could you place it in a pot of boiling water?
2. Cook until tender, about 5 minutes.
3. To make fresh edamame tender, steam them for five to seven minutes.
4. After they are cooked, rinse the edamame and put them in a bowl.
5. To taste, add a sprinkle of sea salt.
6. Present and savor!

BENEFITS:
Rich in fiber, vitamins, and minerals, edamame is a complete protein source that makes a filling and healthy snack.

NUTRITION PLAN: PER SERVING
Calories: 100, Protein: 9g, Carbohydrates: 8g, Fat: 3.5g

SIDE DISHES

VEGETABLE SOUP

COOKING TIME: 30 MINUTES, SERVING: 4 SERVINGS

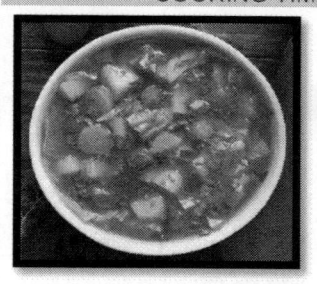

Vegetable soup is a comforting and nutritious dish made by simmering various vegetables in broth, perfect as a side dish or light meal.

INGREDIENTS:
- Assorted vegetables (carrots, celery, onions, zucchini, bell peppers, etc.)
- Vegetable broth
- Herbs and spices (such as thyme, rosemary, bay leaves, salt, and pepper)

STEP-BY-STEP INSTRUCTIONS:
1. Chop all the vegetables into bite-sized pieces.
2. In a large pot, heat some olive oil over medium heat.
3. Add the chopped vegetables to the pot and sauté for a few minutes until they soften.
4. Pour in enough vegetable broth to cover the vegetables.
5. Add herbs and spices according to taste preferences.
6. Bring the soup to a boil, then reduce the heat and let it simmer for about 20-25 minutes until the vegetables are tender.
7. Adjust seasoning if necessary and serve hot.

BENEFITS:

Vegetable soup is low in calories, high in fiber, and packed with essential vitamins and minerals, making it a nutritious addition to any meal.

NUTRITION PLAN: PER SERVING
Calories: 100, Protein: 3g, Carbohydrates: 20g, Fat: 1g

QUINOA PILAF

COOKING TIME: 20 MINUTES, SERVING: 4 SERVINGS

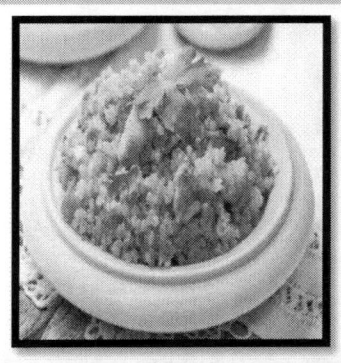

Quinoa pilaf is a flavorful and nutrient-rich side dish made by cooking quinoa with diced vegetables and herbs. Perfect for grilled chicken or fish.

INGREDIENTS:
- Quinoa
- Assorted vegetables (such as carrots, peas, corn, bell peppers, etc.)
- Olive oil
- Garlic
- Vegetable or chicken broth
- Herbs and spices (such as thyme, oregano, salt, and pepper)

STEP-BY-STEP INSTRUCTIONS:
1. Give the quinoa a quick rinse in cold water.
2. Heat a small amount of olive oil in a saucepan over medium heat.
3. When aromatic, add the minced garlic and sauté it.
4. When the vegetables soften, add the diced ones to the saucepan and cook.
5. After rinsing, stir in the quinoa and cook for a short while.
6. Add the chicken or veggie broth and heat until it boils.
7. Once the quinoa is cooked and the liquid has been absorbed, lower the heat, cover, and simmer for 15 to 20 minutes.
8. Using a fork, fluff the quinoa, add the seasoning if needed, and serve hot.

BENEFITS:
Quinoa pilaf helps with digestion and offers long-lasting energy as a gluten-free source of fiber and protein.

NUTRITION PLAN: PER SERVING
Calories: 150, Protein: 5g, Carbohydrates: 25g, Fat: 3g

STEAMED BROCCOLI

COOKING TIME: 15 MINUTES, SERVING: 4 SERVINGS

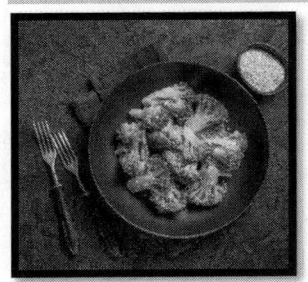

Steaming broccoli till it's crisp-tender is a quick and healthy side dish that tastes great when seasoned with garlic and lemon juice.

INGREDIENTS:
- Broccoli florets
- Water
- Salt
- Lemon juice
- Minced garlic

STEP-BY-STEP INSTRUCTIONS:
1. The broccoli florets should be rinsed under cold water and then patted dry.
2. After bringing a pot of water to a boil, season with salt.
3. After putting the broccoli florets in a colander or steamer basket, place it over the boiling water.
4. Cover the pot and steam the broccoli until soft but still bright green for five to seven minutes.
5. The broccoli should be removed from the steamer and placed on a serving dish.
6. Add a little lemon juice and chopped garlic on top.
7. Gently toss the broccoli to ensure that the seasoning is evenly coated.
8. As a wholesome side dish, serve hot.

BENEFITS:
Steamed broccoli is a low-calorie, high-fiber vegetable that is also strong in vitamins and minerals, such as vitamins K and C, which boost immunity and general health.

NUTRITION PLAN: PER SERVING
Calories: 50, Protein: 3g, Carbohydrates: 10g, Fat: 0.5g

ROASTED BRUSSELS SPROUTS
COOKING TIME: 25 MINUTES, SERVING: 4 SERVINGS

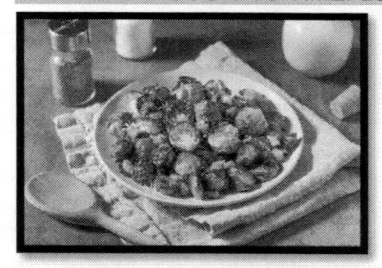

A tasty and fulfilling side dish is made with roasted Brussels sprouts, crispy, caramelized, and seasoned with balsamic vinegar and olive oil.

INGREDIENTS:
- Brussels sprouts
- Olive oil
- Balsamic vinegar
- Salt
- Pepper

STEP-BY-STEP INSTRUCTIONS:
1. Set oven temperature to 400°F or 200°C.
2. Cut the Brussels sprouts in half lengthwise after trimming the ends.
3. Spread some olive oil over the Brussels sprouts placed on a baking pan.
4. To taste, add salt and pepper for seasoning.
5. Toss the Brussels sprouts in the oil and season to coat them evenly.
6. Roast the Brussels sprouts in the oven for 20 to 25 minutes, turning them halfway through or until they are crisp-tender and golden brown.
7. Take it out of the oven and pour some balsamic vinegar over it.
8. Serve hot as a tasty and wholesome side dish.

BENEFITS:
Rich in fiber, vitamins, and antioxidants, roasted Brussels sprouts help to reduce inflammation and promote intestinal health.

NUTRITION PLAN: PER SERVING
Calories: 80, Protein: 4g, Carbohydrates: 10g, Fat: 3g

CAULIFLOWER MASH

COOKING TIME: 20 MINUTES, SERVING: 4 SERVINGS

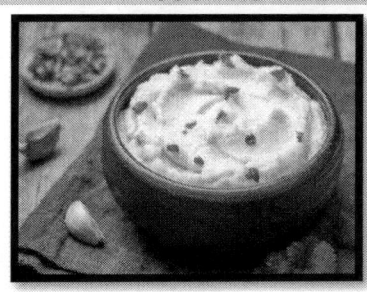

A tasty and creamy side dish, cauliflower mash is produced by boiling cauliflower and then mashing it with butter and seasonings. It's a low-carb substitute for mashed potatoes.

INGREDIENTS:
- [ ] Cauliflower
- [ ] Butter
- [ ] Garlic powder
- [ ] Salt
- [ ] Pepper

STEP-BY-STEP INSTRUCTIONS:
1. After cutting the cauliflower into florets, steam them for 10 to 12 minutes or until they are soft.
2. After draining, add the cauliflower to a food processor.
3. Add butter, salt, pepper, and garlic powder to the food processor.
4. Using a spatula to scrape down the edges as necessary, pulse the cauliflower until smooth and creamy.
5. If needed, adjust the seasoning by tasting it.
6. Top the cauliflower mash with fresh herbs after transferring it to a serving dish.
7. Serve hot as a tasty, lower-carb substitute for mashed potatoes.

BENEFITS:
Mashed cauliflower has a creamy, delicious texture without the added starch of potatoes. It's low in calories and carbs, high in fiber, and full of vitamins.

NUTRITION PLAN: PER SERVING
Calories: 60, Protein: 3g, Carbohydrates: 6g, Fat: 3.5g

MEAL PLAN CHARTS FOR 30 DAYS

S/N	TIME	RECIPES
01	BREAKFAST	Greek Yogurt Parfait
01	LUNCH	Turkey Lettuce Wraps
01	DINNER	Baked Salmon
01	SNACK	Almonds, Apple Slices with Peanut Butter
01	SIDE DISH	Steamed Broccoli
02	BREAKFAST	Veggie Omelette
02	LUNCH	Quinoa Salad
02	DINNER	Turkey Meatballs
02	SNACK	Baby Carrots and Hummus, Cottage Cheese with Pineapple
02	SIDE DISH	Quinoa Pilaf
03	BREAKFAST	Protein Pancakes
03	LUNCH	Veggie Stir-Fry
03	DINNER	Stir-Fried Tofu
03	SNACK	Hard-boiled eggs, Celery Sticks with Almond Butter
03	SIDE DISH	Roasted Brussels Sprouts
04	BREAKFAST	Avocado Toast
04	LUNCH	Tuna Salad

	DINNER	Chicken Stir-Fry
	SNACK	Edamame, Greek Yogurt
	SIDE DISH	Cauliflower Mash
05	BREAKFAST	Breakfast Burrito
	LUNCH	Lentil Soup
	DINNER	Grilled Veggie Skewers
	SNACK	Almonds, Chia Seed Pudding
	SIDE DISH	Vegetable Soup
06	BREAKFAST	Overnight Oats
	LUNCH	Quinoa Bowl
	DINNER	Spaghetti Squash with Marinara
	SNACK	Apple Slices with Peanut Butter, Baby Carrots and Hummus
	SIDE DISH	Cauliflower Fried Rice
07	BREAKFAST	Smoothie Bowl
	LUNCH	Stuffed Bell Peppers
	DINNER	Turkey Chili
	SNACK	Greek Yogurt, Celery Sticks with Almond Butter
	SIDE DISH	Quinoa Pilaf
08	BREAKFAST	Veggie Omelette
	LUNCH	Turkey Lettuce Wraps
	DINNER	Baked Salmon
	SNACK	Almonds, Apple Slices with Peanut Butter
	SIDE DISH	Steamed Broccoli
09	BREAKFAST	Greek Yogurt Parfait
	LUNCH	Quinoa Salad
	DINNER	Turkey Meatballs
	SNACK	Baby Carrots and Hummus, Cottage Cheese with Pineapple
	SIDE DISH	Quinoa Pilaf
10	BREAKFAST	Protein Pancakes
	LUNCH	Veggie Stir-Fry
	DINNER	Stir-Fried Tofu
	SNACK	Hard-boiled eggs, Celery Sticks with Almond Butter
	SIDE DISH	Roasted Brussels Sprouts
11	BREAKFAST	Avocado Toast
	LUNCH	Tuna Salad
	DINNER	Chicken Stir-Fry
	SNACK	Edamame, Greek Yogurt
	SIDE DISH	Cauliflower Mash
12	BREAKFAST	Breakfast Burrito
	LUNCH	Lentil Soup
	DINNER	Grilled Veggie Skewers
	SNACK	Almonds, Chia Seed Pudding
	SIDE DISH	Vegetable Soup
13	BREAKFAST	Overnight Oats
	LUNCH	Quinoa Bowl
	DINNER	Spaghetti Squash with Marinara
	SNACK	Apple Slices with Peanut Butter, Baby Carrots and Hummus
	SIDE DISH	Cauliflower Fried Rice
14	BREAKFAST	Smoothie Bowl
	LUNCH	Stuffed Bell Peppers
	DINNER	Turkey Chili
	SNACK	Greek Yogurt, Celery Sticks with Almond Butter
	SIDE DISH	Quinoa Pilaf

Day	Meal	Dish
15	BREAKFAST	Veggie Omelette
	LUNCH	Turkey Lettuce Wraps
	DINNER	Baked Salmon
	SNACK	Almonds, Apple Slices with Peanut Butter
	SIDE DISH	Steamed Broccoli
16	BREAKFAST	Greek Yogurt Parfait
	LUNCH	Quinoa Salad
	DINNER	Turkey Meatballs
	SNACK	Baby Carrots and Hummus, Cottage Cheese with Pineapple
	SIDE DISH	Quinoa Pilaf
17	BREAKFAST	Protein Pancakes
	LUNCH	Veggie Stir-Fry
	DINNER	Stir-Fried Tofu
	SNACK	Hard-boiled eggs, Celery Sticks with Almond Butter
	SIDE DISH	Roasted Brussels Sprouts
18	BREAKFAST	Avocado Toast
	LUNCH	Tuna Salad
	DINNER	Chicken Stir-Fry
	SNACK	Edamame, Greek Yogurt
	SIDE DISH	Cauliflower Mash
19	BREAKFAST	Breakfast Burrito
	LUNCH	Lentil Soup
	DINNER	Grilled Veggie Skewers
	SNACK	Almonds, Chia Seed Pudding
	SIDE DISH	Vegetable Soup
20	BREAKFAST	Overnight Oats
	LUNCH	Quinoa Bowl
	DINNER	Spaghetti Squash with Marinara
	SNACK	Apple Slices with Peanut Butter, Baby Carrots and Hummus
	SIDE DISH	Cauliflower Fried Rice
21	BREAKFAST	Smoothie Bowl
	LUNCH	Stuffed Bell Peppers
	DINNER	Turkey Chili
	SNACK	Greek Yogurt, Celery Sticks with Almond Butter
	SIDE DISH	Quinoa Pilaf
22	BREAKFAST	Veggie Omelette
	LUNCH	Turkey Lettuce Wraps
	DINNER	Baked Salmon
	SNACK	Almonds, Apple Slices with Peanut Butter
	SIDE DISH	Steamed Broccoli
23	BREAKFAST	Greek Yogurt Parfait
	LUNCH	Quinoa Salad
	DINNER	Turkey Meatballs
	SNACK	Baby Carrots and Hummus, Cottage Cheese with Pineapple
	SIDE DISH	Quinoa Pilaf
24	BREAKFAST	Protein Pancakes
	LUNCH	Veggie Stir-Fry
	DINNER	Stir-Fried Tofu
	SNACK	Hard-boiled eggs, Celery Sticks with Almond Butter
	SIDE DISH	Roasted Brussels Sprouts
25	BREAKFAST	Avocado Toast
	LUNCH	Tuna Salad
	DINNER	Chicken Stir-Fry

	SNACK	Edamame, Greek Yogurt
	SIDE DISH	Cauliflower Mash
26	BREAKFAST	Breakfast Burrito
	LUNCH	Lentil Soup
	DINNER	Grilled Veggie Skewers
	SNACK	Almonds, Chia Seed Pudding
	SIDE DISH	Vegetable Soup
27	BREAKFAST	Overnight Oats
	LUNCH	Quinoa Bowl
	DINNER	Spaghetti Squash with Marinara
	SNACK	Apple Slices with Peanut Butter, Baby Carrots and Hummus
	SIDE DISH	Cauliflower Fried Rice
28	BREAKFAST	Smoothie Bowl
	LUNCH	Stuffed Bell Peppers
	DINNER	Turkey Chili
	SNACK	Greek Yogurt, Celery Sticks with Almond Butter
	SIDE DISH	Quinoa Pilaf
29	BREAKFAST	Veggie Omelette
	LUNCH	Turkey Lettuce Wraps
	DINNER	Baked Salmon
	SNACK	Almonds, Apple Slices with Peanut Butter
	SIDE DISH	Steamed Broccoli
30	BREAKFAST	Greek Yogurt Parfait
	LUNCH	Quinoa Salad
	DINNER	Turkey Meatballs
	SNACK	Baby Carrots and Hummus, Cottage Cheese with Pineapple
	SIDE DISH	Quinoa Pilaf

DR. NOWZARADAN'S MEAL PLAN ON A BUDGET

"Dr. Nowzaradan's Meal Plan on a Budget" is now open! This book offers doable tactics and inexpensive dinner ideas to help you reach your weight loss objectives without exceeding the budget. Dr. Nowzaradan's weight loss strategy emphasizes portion control and a balanced diet; with some preparation and ingenuity, you may adhere to his recommendations without exceeding budget.

INTRODUCTION

"Dr. Nowzaradan's Meal Plan on a Budget" Eating wholesome, affordable meals while adhering to a strict budget might be difficult. However, you can reach your weight loss objectives without breaking if you have the correct plans and direction. This book is your go-to resource for understanding how to prepare meals on a tight budget while following the guidelines of Dr. Nowzaradan's well-known weight loss program.

Dr. Nowzaradan's concept emphasizes the importance of sustainable lifestyle changes, portion control, and a balanced diet. Implementing these ideas into our meal plans without sacrificing flavor or quality may significantly reduce our body weight and enhance our general health.

BREAKFAST RECIPES

OATMEAL WITH BANANA SLICES

COOKING TIME: 10 MINUTES, SERVING: 1 SERVING

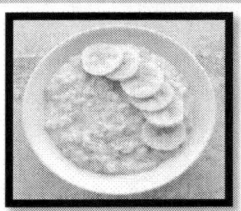

oatmeal cooked with milk or water and banana slices on top. It's an inexpensive, wholesome, high-fiber, high-potassium breakfast choice.

INGREDIENTS:
- 1/2 cup oats
- 1 cup water or milk
- One banana, sliced

STEP-BY-STEP INSTRUCTIONS:
1. Heat the milk or water in a small pot until it boils.
2. After adding the oats, turn the heat down to medium.
3. Cook until thickened, stirring regularly, for 5 minutes with the oats.
4. Take it off the stove and give it a minute to rest.
5. Once the oatmeal is in a bowl, cover it with sliced banana.
6. Enjoy while hot!

BENEFITS:
Bananas supply potassium and naturally occurring sweetness without additional sugar, while oatmeal offers complex carbohydrates and fiber for long-lasting energy.

NUTRITION PLAN: PER SERVING
Calories: 250, Protein: 5g, Carbohydrates: 52g, Fat: 3g

EGG MUFFINS

COOKING TIME: 25 MINUTES, SERVING: 6 MUFFINS

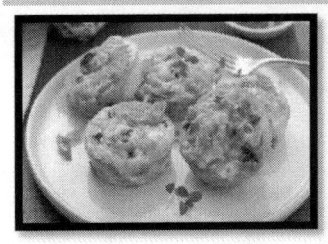

Eggs baked with chopped vegetables in muffin tins provide a portable, high-protein breakfast choice.

INGREDIENTS:
- Six eggs
- 1/4 cup diced bell peppers
- 1/4 cup diced onions
- 1/4 cup diced spinach
- Salt and pepper to taste

STEP-BY-STEP INSTRUCTIONS:
1. Set a muffin tin to 350°F (175°C) and preheat the oven.
2. Mix eggs, chopped veggies, salt, and pepper in a bowl.
3. Spoon the egg mixture into each muffin tray, filling it to about three-quarters of the way.
4. Cook the egg muffins for 20 to 25 minutes until they are set and have a hint of color on top.
5. Let them cool a little before taking them out of the muffin tray.
6. Warm food can be served or refrigerated for later use.

BENEFITS:
Egg muffins are a quick, adaptable breakfast choice, packed with protein and other nutrients from veggies.

NUTRITION PLAN: PER SERVING
Calories: 80, Protein: 7g, Carbohydrates: 2g, Fat: 5g

YOGURT WITH GRANOLA

COOKING TIME: 5 MINUTES, SERVING: 1 BOWL

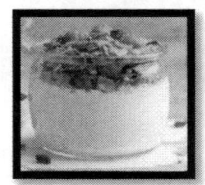

A straightforward and affordable breakfast option is plain yogurt with store-bought or homemade granola.

INGREDIENTS:
- 1/2 cup plain yogurt
- 1/4 cup granola

STEP-BY-STEP INSTRUCTIONS:
1. Pour the yogurt into a bowl using a spoon.
2. Over the yogurt, scatter the granola.
3. Enjoy and serve right away.

BENEFITS:
This breakfast is filling and healthy because it has a decent protein, healthy fats, and carbohydrate ratio.

NUTRITION PLAN: PER SERVING
Calories: 200, Protein: 9g, Carbohydrates: 30g, Fat: 6g

BREAKFAST QUESADILLA

COOKING TIME: 10 MINUTES, SERVING: 1 QUESADILLA

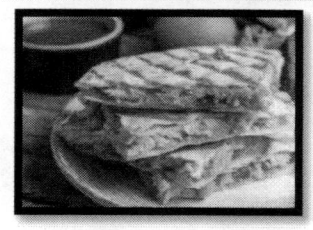

A satisfying and reasonably priced breakfast is a whole grain tortilla stuffed with scrambled eggs, cheese, and salsa.

INGREDIENTS:
- One whole-grain tortilla
- Two eggs scrambled
- 1/4 cup shredded cheese
- Two tablespoons salsa

STEP-BY-STEP INSTRUCTIONS:
1. A non-stick skillet should be heated to medium heat.
2. Warm the tortilla for one or two minutes in the skillet.
3. Using half of the tortilla, evenly distribute the scrambled eggs.
4. Over the eggs, scatter the grated cheese.
5. To cover the filling, fold the tortilla in half.
6. Cook the tortilla for two to three more minutes, turning it halfway through or until the cheese is melted and golden brown.
7. After removing from the skillet, cut into wedges.
8. Present the salsa separately.

BENEFITS:
Packed with protein and fiber, this breakfast will keep you content and full until your next meal.

NUTRITION PLAN: PER SERVING
Calories: 350, Protein: 21g, Carbohydrates: 24g, Fat: 18g

AVOCADO TOAST WITH HARD-BOILED EGG

COOKING TIME: 15 MINUTES, SERVING: 1 SERVING

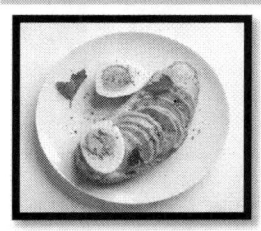

This recipe offers a low-cost and high-protein breakfast option. It consists of whole-grain toast with sliced hard-boiled egg and mashed avocado.

INGREDIENTS:
- One slice whole grain bread toasted
- 1/2 ripe avocado, mashed
- One hard-boiled egg, sliced

STEP-BY-STEP INSTRUCTIONS:
1. When the whole grain bread is golden brown, toast it.
2. In a small bowl, mash the avocado with a fork until it's smooth.
3. Over the toast, equally, distribute the mashed avocado.
4. Place the hard-boiled egg slices over the avocado.
5. If desired, season with salt and pepper to taste.
6. Serve right away.

BENEFITS:
Packed with fiber, protein, and healthy fats, this breakfast will keep you full and energized all morning.

NUTRITION PLAN: PER SERVING
Calories: 280, Protein: 13g, Carbohydrates: 20g, Fat: 17g

LUNCH RECIPES

BLACK BEAN QUESADILLAS

COOKING TIME: 15 MINUTES, SERVING: MAKES 2 QUESADILLAS

Black bean quesadillas are a satisfying and affordable lunch option

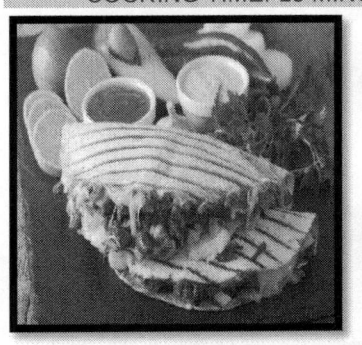

INGREDIENTS:
- Four whole-grain tortillas
- One can (15 oz) black beans, drained
- 1 cup shredded cheese (cheddar, Monterey Jack, or Mexican blend)

OPTIONAL TOPPINGS:
- Salsa
- Avocado
- Greek yogurt

STEP-BY-STEP INSTRUCTIONS:
1. A non-stick skillet should be heated to medium heat.
2. Use a fork to mash the black beans in a bowl until they are smooth.
3. Spread half of the mashed black beans equally over half of the tortilla after placing it in the skillet.
4. Top the black beans with half of the shredded cheese.
5. To form a half-moon, fold the remaining tortilla over the filling.
6. Cook until brown and crispy, 2 to 3 minutes per side.

7. Continue with the remaining tortillas and the components for the filling.
8. Serve the quesadillas hot with optional toppings after slicing them into wedges.

BENEFITS:
Black bean quesadillas are a filling and healthy lunch option because they contain fantastic fiber and plant-based protein.

NUTRITION PLAN: PER QUESADILLA
Calories: 300, Protein: 15g, Carbohydrates: 30g, Fat: 10g

QUINOA SALAD WITH VEGGIES
COOKING TIME: 20 MINUTES, SERVING: MAKES 4 SERVINGS

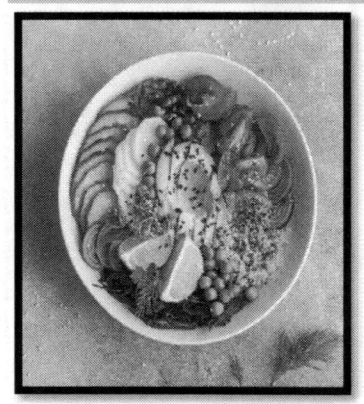

A cheap and healthy lunch option is a quinoa salad with veggies consisting of cooked quinoa, chopped vegetables, and a primary vinaigrette dressing.

INGREDIENTS:
- 1 cup quinoa, rinsed
- 2 cups water or vegetable broth
- One cucumber, diced
- One bell pepper, diced
- 1 cup cherry tomatoes, halved
- 1/4 cup red onion, finely chopped
- 1/4 cup fresh parsley, chopped
- Juice of 1 lemon
- Two tablespoons of olive oil
- Salt and pepper to taste

STEP-BY-STEP INSTRUCTIONS:
1. Bring the vegetable broth or water to a boil in a medium saucepan. After adding the quinoa, lower the heat to a simmer, cover, and let the quinoa cook for 15 to 20 minutes or until the water has been absorbed. Turn off the heat and let it cool.
2. Cooked quinoa, sliced cucumber, bell pepper, cherry tomatoes, red onion, and chopped parsley should all be combined in a big bowl.
3. To create the dressing, combine the lemon juice, olive oil, salt, and pepper in a small bowl.
4. After adding the dressing, toss the quinoa salad to ensure an even coating.
5. Serve at either room temperature or cold.

BENEFITS:
Quinoa salad supports weight loss attempts and general health by offering a balanced combination of protein, fiber, vitamins, and minerals.

NUTRITION PLAN: PER SERVING
Calories: 200, Protein: 5g, Carbohydrates: 30g, Fat: 8g

RICE AND BEAN BOWL

COOKING TIME: 30 MINUTES, SERVING: MAKES 4 SERVINGS

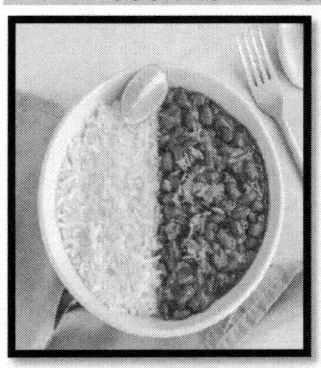

A satisfying and reasonably priced lunch option is a rice and bean bowl, which combines cooked rice with chopped tomatoes, canned beans, and avocado slices.

INGREDIENTS:
- [ ] 1 cup long-grain rice
- [ ] 2 cups water or vegetable broth
- [ ] One can (15 oz) black beans
- [ ] 1 cup diced tomatoes
- [ ] One avocado, sliced
- [ ] 1/4 cup chopped cilantro
- [ ] Juice of 1 lime
- [ ] Salt and pepper to taste

STEP-BY-STEP INSTRUCTIONS:
1. Bring the vegetable broth or water to a boil in a medium saucepan. When the rice is soft and the water has been absorbed, add the rice, lower the heat to low, cover, and simmer for 18 to 20 minutes. After turning off the heat, leave it for five minutes.
2. Cooked rice, black beans, diced tomatoes, avocado slices, and chopped cilantro should all be combined in a big bowl.
3. Add salt and pepper to taste, and squeeze the lime juice over the rice and bean combination.
4. Mix everything until thoroughly incorporated.
5. Heat or serve at room temperature.

BENEFITS:
A rice and bean bowl is a filling and healthy dinner option since it offers a balanced combination of healthy fats, protein, and carbohydrates.

NUTRITION PLAN: PER SERVING
Calories: 300, Protein: 10g, Carbohydrates: 50g, Fat: 8g

PASTA PRIMAVERA

COOKING TIME: 25 MINUTES, SERVING: MAKES 4 SERVINGS

A tasty and reasonably priced lunch choice is spaghetti primavera,

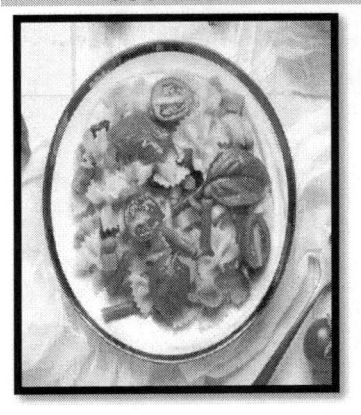

INGREDIENTS:
- [ ] 8 oz whole wheat pasta
- [ ] 2 tbsp olive oil
- [ ] Two cloves garlic, minced
- [ ] One small onion, diced
- [ ] One bell pepper, thinly sliced
- [ ] One zucchini, diced
- [ ] 1 cup cherry tomatoes, halved
- [ ] 1 cup marinara sauce
- [ ] Salt and pepper to taste
- [ ] Fresh basil leaves for garnish (optional)

STEP-BY-STEP INSTRUCTIONS:
1. Pasta should be cooked as directed on the package until it is al dente. After draining, set away.
2. Heat the olive oil in a large skillet over medium heat. Add the onion and minced garlic, and sauté until they are transparent and fragrant.
3. Add the diced zucchini and the sliced bell pepper to the skillet. Simmer the veggies for five to seven minutes or until they are soft.
4. Add the cherry tomatoes halves and simmer for two to three minutes.
5. Add the marinara sauce and cooked pasta to the skillet. Mix everything until the sauce coats the pasta and veggies equally.
6. To taste, add salt and pepper for seasoning.
7. If preferred, top the heated Pasta Primavera with fresh basil leaves.

BENEFITS:
A tasty and filling lunch choice, pasta primavera offers a good mix of carbs, fiber, vitamins, and minerals.

NUTRITION PLAN: PER SERVING
Calories: 350, Protein: 10g, Carbohydrates: 60g, Fat: 8g

DINNER RECIPES

SPAGHETTI AGLIO E OLIO

COOKING TIME: 20 MINUTES, SERVING: MAKES 4 SERVINGS

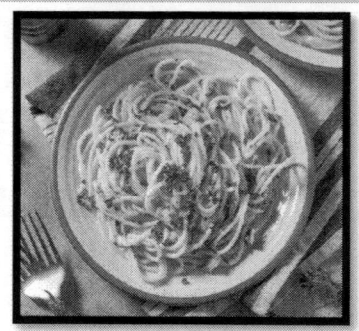

A famous Italian pasta dish called spaghetti aglio e olio consists of spaghetti mixed with olive oil infused with garlic, red pepper flakes, and parsley for a tasty and easy dinner.

INGREDIENTS:
- 8 oz spaghetti
- 1/4 cup olive oil
- Four cloves garlic, thinly sliced
- 1/2 tsp red pepper flakes (adjust to taste)
- Salt and pepper to taste
- 2 tbsp chopped fresh parsley

STEP-BY-STEP INSTRUCTIONS:
1. Cook the pasta until al dente, following the directions on the package. After draining, set away.
2. Heat the olive oil in a large skillet over medium heat. Add the sliced garlic and red pepper flakes and simmer for two to three minutes or until the garlic is aromatic and golden.
3. When the spaghetti is done, add it to the skillet and toss it to coat it uniformly with the garlic-scented oil. To taste, add salt and pepper for seasoning.
4. Top the spaghetti with the chopped parsley after taking the skillet off the burner.
5. Garnish the hot spaghetti Aglio e Olio with more parsley, if preferred.

BENEFITS:
This meal is a light and filling alternative for dinner because it is low in calories and healthy fats from olive oil.

NUTRITION PLAN: PER SERVING

Calories: 250-300, Protein: 6-8g, Carbohydrates: 30-35g, Fat: 10-12g

BAKED CHICKEN DRUMSTICKS

COOKING TIME: 45 MINUTES, SERVING: MAKES 4 SERVINGS

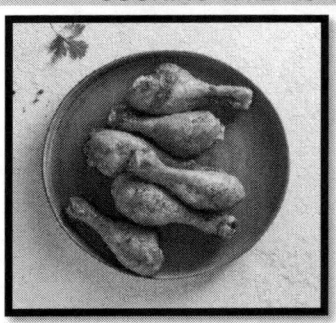

A cheap and high-protein supper option is roasted chicken drumsticks seasoned with herbs and spices and baked till golden brown.

INGREDIENTS:
- Eight chicken drumsticks
- 2 tbsp olive oil
- 1 tsp paprika
- 1 tsp garlic powder
- 1 tsp onion powder
- 1/2 tsp dried thyme
- Salt and pepper to taste

STEP-BY-STEP INSTRUCTIONS:
1. Set oven temperature to 400°F or 200°C. Cover a baking sheet with foil or parchment paper.
2. In a small bowl, combine the olive oil, paprika, dried thyme, onion and garlic powders, salt, and pepper.
3. Paint dry the chicken drumsticks using paper towels, then coat them thoroughly with the seasoned olive oil mixture.
4. Place the chicken drumsticks on the baking sheet prepared in a single layer.
5. Bake for 35 to 40 minutes in a preheated oven or until the chicken is thoroughly cooked and the skin is crispy and browned.
6. Before serving, take the chicken out of the oven and rest for a few minutes.

BENEFITS:
Seasoned with herbs and spices for flavor without adding unnecessary calories, baked chicken drumsticks are a lean source of protein.

NUTRITION PLAN: PER SERVING
Calories: 150-200, Protein: 20-25g, Carbohydrates: 0g, Fat: 8-10g

ONE-POT CHILI

COOKING TIME: 1 HOUR, SERVING: MAKES 6 SERVINGS

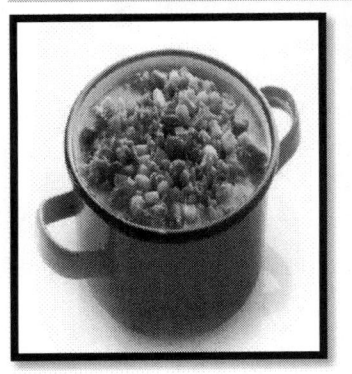

A filling and tasty chili that can be made on a budget.

INGREDIENTS:
- 1 lb (450g) lean ground beef or turkey
- One onion, diced
- Three cloves garlic, minced
- One bell pepper, diced
- One can (14 oz/400g) diced tomatoes
- 2 cups (480ml) beef or vegetable broth
- 2 tbsp chili powder
- 1 tsp cumin
- 1 tsp paprika
- Salt and pepper to taste

STEP-BY-STEP INSTRUCTIONS:
1. Brown the ground beef or turkey in a big pot or Dutch oven over medium heat. If necessary, drain the extra fat.
2. Add the diced bell pepper, diced onion, and minced garlic to the pot. Simmer the veggies for five to seven minutes or until they are tender.
3. Add the chopped tomatoes, kidney beans (drained and rinsed), black beans, chili powder, cumin, paprika, beef or vegetable broth, and salt and pepper.
4. After bringing the chili to a simmer, lower the heat and cover it. Cook, stirring now and again, for 30 to 40 minutes or until the flavors are fully blended and the consistency of the chili is to your liking.
5. If necessary, taste and adjust the seasoning. On top, serve hot with your preferred toppings (shredded cheese, chopped green onions, sour cream, etc.).

BENEFITS:
This one-pot chili is a hearty and fulfilling supper packed with protein, fiber, and essential nutrients from various beans and vegetables.

NUTRITION PLAN: PER SERVING
Calories: 250-300, Protein: 15-20g, Carbohydrates: 20-25g, Fat: 10-15g

STUFFED BELL PEPPERS WITH RICE AND BEANS

COOKING TIME: 1 HOUR, SERVING: MAKES 4 SERVINGS

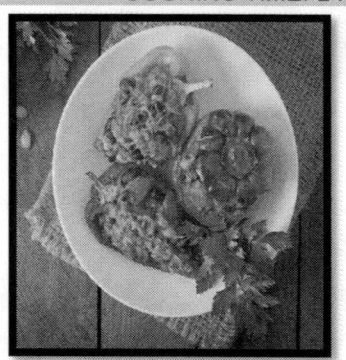

A filling and reasonably priced supper choice

INGREDIENTS:
- Four large bell peppers (any color),
- 1 cup (200g) cooked brown rice
- 1 cup (150g) corn kernels (fresh, frozen)
- One onion, diced
- Two cloves garlic, minced
- One can (14 oz/400g) diced tomatoes
- 1 tsp cumin
- 1 tsp chili powder
- Salt and pepper to taste
- Shredded cheese for topping (optional)

STEP-BY-STEP INSTRUCTIONS:
1. Turn the oven on to 375°F, or 190°C. Place the bell pepper halves cut side up in a baking dish.
2. Heat olive oil in a large skillet over medium heat. Add the minced garlic and chopped onion and cook until tender.
3. Add chopped tomatoes (with their liquids), black beans, corn kernels, cumin, chili powder, salt, and pepper to the skillet. Cook, stirring constantly, for a few minutes until thoroughly heated.
4. Fill half the bell pepper with a spoonful of the rice and bean mixture.
5. Bake the baking dish in the oven for thirty to thirty-five minutes, or until the peppers are soft, covered with aluminum foil.
6. Remove the foil, top each stuffed pepper with shredded cheese, if desired, and bake for five minutes or until the cheese is bubbling and melted.
7. If preferred, top with fresh herbs like parsley or cilantro and serve hot.

BENEFITS:

Packed with fiber, protein, and vital minerals from the beans, veggies, and whole grains, these stuffed bell peppers are a hearty and filling dinner that fits well with Dr. Nowzaradan's diet plan.

NUTRITION PLAN: PER SERVING
Calories: 200-250, Protein: 8-10g, Carbohydrates: 30-35g, Fat: 5-7g

BAKED FISH FILLETS

COOKING TIME: 25 MINUTES, SERVING: MAKES 4 SERVINGS

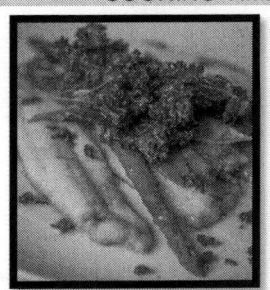

Seasoned fish fillets baked with lemon juice and herbs until flaky and tender, providing a protein-rich and budget-friendly dinner option.

INGREDIENTS:
- Four fish fillets (such as tilapia, cod, or salmon)
- 2 tbsp olive oil
- 2 tbsp lemon juice
- Two cloves garlic, minced
- 1 tsp dried herbs (such as thyme, oregano)
- Salt and pepper to taste

STEP-BY-STEP INSTRUCTIONS:
1. Turn the oven on to 375°F, or 190°C. Cover a baking sheet with foil or parchment paper.
2. After the baking sheet is ready, put the fish fillets on it.
3. In a small bowl, mix the olive oil, lemon juice, dried herbs, minced garlic, salt, and pepper.
4. Evenly coat the fish fillets by brushing them with the mixture.
5. Fish should be baked for 15 to 20 minutes in a preheated oven or until it is opaque and flakes readily with a fork.
6. If preferred, top with slices of lemon or fresh herbs and serve hot.

BENEFITS:
This recipe is a wholesome and filling choice for Dr. Nowzaradan's diet plan because it has a lean source of protein from the fish and healthy fats from the olive oil.

NUTRITION PLAN: PER SERVING
Calories: 150-200, Protein: 20-25g, Carbohydrates: 0g, Fat: 8-10g

VEGETABLE PASTA BAKE

COOKING TIME: 40 MINUTES, SERVING: MAKES 6 SERVINGS

A comforting and budget-friendly dinner option,

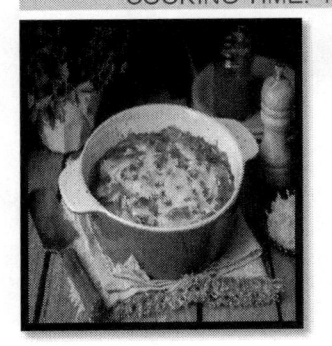

INGREDIENTS:
- 8 oz (about 225g) whole wheat pasta
- 1 tbsp olive oil
- One onion, diced
- Two cloves garlic, minced
- Two bell peppers and One zucchini, diced
- 1 cup mushrooms, sliced
- 2 cups marinara sauce
- 1 cup shredded cheese
- Salt and pepper to taste

STEP-BY-STEP INSTRUCTIONS:
1. Turn the oven on to 375°F, or 190°C. Pasta should be cooked as directed on the package until it is al dente. After draining, set away.
2. Heat the olive oil in a big skillet over medium heat. Add the chopped onion and garlic, and simmer for two to three minutes or until softened and aromatic.
3. Add the chopped bell peppers, mushrooms, and zucchini to the skillet—Sauté the vegetables for five to seven minutes or until soft. To taste, add salt and pepper for seasoning.
4. Stir the cooked pasta and marinara sauce together thoroughly in the skillet.
5. Spoon the mixture into a baking dish that has been buttered. Evenly distribute cheese shreds on top.
6. In a preheated oven, bake for 20 to 25 minutes or until the cheese is bubbling and melted.
7. If preferred, top with freshly chopped herbs and serve hot.

BENEFITS:
This meal is a filling and healthy supper alternative for Dr. Nowzaradan's diet plan since it balances carbohydrates, protein, and veggies.

NUTRITION PLAN: PER SERVING
Calories: 250-300, Protein: 10-15g, Carbohydrates: 30-40g, Fat: 8-10g

BEAN AND VEGETABLE CASSEROLE
COOKING TIME: 1 HOUR, SERVING: MAKES 8 SERVINGS

It's bubbling and tasty is a healthy and inexpensive supper option.

INGREDIENTS:
- Two cans (15 oz each) of beans
- One onion, diced
- Two cloves garlic, minced
- Two bell peppers diced
- Two zucchinis, diced
- 1 cup corn kernels (fresh, frozen, or canned)
- 2 cups tomato sauce
- 1 cup shredded cheese
- Salt and pepper to taste

STEP-BY-STEP INSTRUCTIONS:
1. Turn the oven on to 375°F, or 190°C. Use cooking spray or olive oil to grease a baking dish.
2. Heat olive oil in a large skillet over medium heat. Add the chopped onion and garlic, and simmer for two to three minutes or until softened and aromatic.
3. Add the chopped zucchini and bell peppers to the skillet—Sauté the vegetables for five to seven minutes or until soft. To taste, add salt and pepper for seasoning.
4. Add the drained beans, tomato sauce, and corn kernels to the sautéed veggies in a mixing bowl. Blend until thoroughly blended.
5. Spoon the batter into the ready baking dish. Evenly distribute it.
6. Top the mixture with cheese that has been shredded.
7. Bake the baking dish for thirty minutes in a preheated oven covered with aluminum foil.

8. After removing the foil, bake for ten to fifteen more minutes or until the cheese is bubbling and melted.
9. Before serving, allow the dish to cool somewhat. Have fun!

BENEFITS:
The doctor finds this casserole a filling and healthy supper option because it's high in fiber, protein, and vital nutrients from the beans and veggies. Nowzaradan's diet plan.

NUTRITION PLAN: PER SERVING
Calories: 200-250, Protein: 8-10g, Carbohydrates: 25-30g, Fat: 6-8g

SNACKS

POPCORN: AIR-POPPED POPCORN WITH HERBS OR NUTRITIONAL YEAST

COOKING TIME: 10 MINUTES, SERVING: MAKES 4 SERVINGS

Air-popped popcorn is a tasty and nutritious snack that is affordable.

INGREDIENTS:
- 1/2 cup popcorn kernels
- 1-2 tsp olive oil or cooking spray
- 1 tsp dried herbs (such as rosemary, thyme, or oregano) or 2 tbsp nutritional yeast
- Salt to taste

STEP-BY-STEP INSTRUCTIONS:
1. As directed by your air popper's instructions, air-pop the popcorn kernels.
2. After popping, move the popcorn to a big bowl.
3. To help the seasoning stay, lightly sprinkle olive oil or mist with cooking spray.
4. Add salt to taste and dried herbs or nutritional yeast to the popcorn, tossing well to apply the spice evenly; toss.
5. Enjoy and serve right away.

BENEFITS:
Popcorn that has been air-popped is a high-fiber, low-calorie snack that keeps you satisfied without packing on the calories.

NUTRITION PLAN: PER SERVING
Calories: 100, Protein: 3g, Carbohydrates: 20g, Fat: 2g

CARROT STICKS WITH HUMMUS

COOKING TIME: 10 MINUTES, SERVING: MAKES 4 SERVINGS

A cheap, high-fiber, high-protein snack packed with nutrients is crunchy carrot sticks and hummus.

INGREDIENTS:
- Four large carrots peeled and cut into sticks
- 1 cup hummus

STEP-BY-STEP INSTRUCTIONS:

1. After peeling, chop the carrots into sticks.
2. Present the carrot sticks alongside a dish of hummus for dunks.

BENEFITS:
This snack's carrots are high in fiber, vitamins, and minerals; the hummus adds protein and good fats.

NUTRITION PLAN: PER SERVING
Calories: 100, Protein: 3g, Carbohydrates: 12g, Fat: 5g

RICE CAKES WITH ALMOND BUTTER

COOKING TIME: 5 MINUTES, SERVING: MAKES 4 SERVINGS

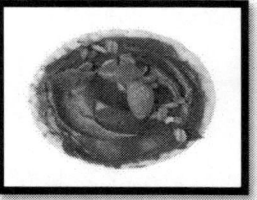

Almond butter-topped rice cakes are a cheap, tasty, and crunchy snack that is simple to make.

INGREDIENTS:
- Four rice cakes
- 4 tbsp almond butter

STEP-BY-STEP INSTRUCTIONS:
1. On each rice cake, spread one spoonful of almond butter.
2. Serve right away.

BENEFITS:
This snack helps to keep you feeling full and content because it is a beautiful dose of protein and healthy fats.

NUTRITION PLAN: PER SERVING
Calories: 150, Protein: 4g, Carbohydrates: 15g, Fat: 9g

TRAIL MIX

COOKING TIME: 5 MINUTES, SERVING: MAKES 4 SERVINGS

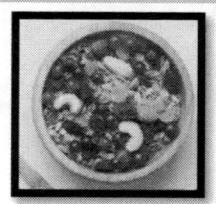

A wholesome and transportable snack is a homemade trail mix, which combines nuts, seeds, and dried fruit.

INGREDIENTS:
- 1/2 cup almonds
- 1/2 cup walnuts
- 1/2 cup sunflower seeds
- 1/2 cup raisins or dried cranberries

STEP-BY-STEP INSTRUCTIONS:
1. Almonds, walnuts, sunflower seeds, and dried fruit should all be combined in a bowl.
2. Stir thoroughly and divide into four portions.

BENEFITS:
Packed with fiber, protein, and healthy fats, this food gives you long-lasting energy and satisfaction.

NUTRITION PLAN: PER SERVING
Calories: 200, Protein: 6g, Carbohydrates: 20g, Fat: 12g

SIDE DISHES

ROASTED VEGETABLES

COOKING TIME: 30 MINUTES, SERVING: MAKES 4 SERVINGS

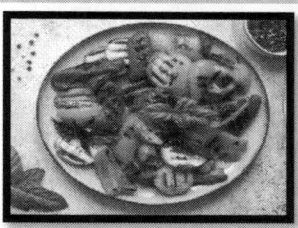

Vegetables become naturally sweet when roasted, which makes this a cost-effective and wholesome side dish.

INGREDIENTS:
- 2 cups diced vegetables (carrots, bell peppers, zucchini, etc.)
- 2 tbsp olive oil
- Salt and pepper to taste

STEP-BY-STEP INSTRUCTIONS:
1. Set oven temperature to 400°F or 200°C.
2. Add salt, pepper, and olive oil to the chopped vegetables and toss.
3. Arrange on a baking sheet in a single layer.
4. Roast for 20 to 25 minutes, tossing occasionally, or until soft and beginning to brown.

BENEFITS:
Packed with vitamins and minerals, this dish also has a lot of fiber.

NUTRITION PLAN: PER SERVING
Calories: 100, Protein: 2g, Carbohydrates: 10g, Fat: 7g

BLACK BEAN SALAD

COOKING TIME: 10 MINUTES, SERVING: MAKES 4 SERVINGS

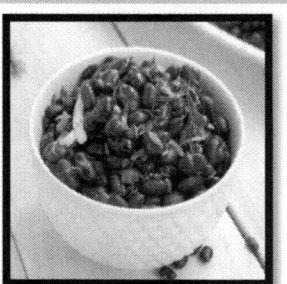

This black bean salad is a simple, low-cost, high-protein side dish that comes together quickly.

INGREDIENTS:
- One can of black beans
- One bell pepper, diced
- One small red onion, diced
- 1 cup corn kernels (fresh or canned)
- 2 tbsp olive oil
- 1 tbsp vinegar
- Salt and pepper to taste

STEP-BY-STEP INSTRUCTIONS:
1. Combine the bell pepper, red onion, corn, and black beans in a bowl.
2. Toss to coat after drizzling with vinegar and olive oil.
3. To taste, add salt and pepper for seasoning.

BENEFITS:
This salad's high fiber and protein content encourages fullness and good digestive health.

NUTRITION PLAN: PER SERVING
Calories: 150, Protein: 7g, Carbohydrates: 25g, Fat: 5g

MASHED SWEET POTATOES

COOKING TIME: 20 MINUTES, SERVING: MAKES 4 SERVINGS

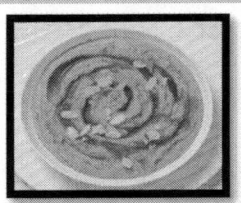

Mashed sweet potatoes with cinnamon and milk are a cheap and healthy side dish.

INGREDIENTS:
- ☐ Two large sweet potatoes, peeled and diced
- ☐ 1/4 cup milk (dairy or non-dairy)
- ☐ 1 tsp cinnamon

STEP-BY-STEP INSTRUCTIONS:
1. Sweet potatoes should be boiled or steamed for about 15 minutes or until soft.
2. After draining, mash till smooth with milk and cinnamon.

BENEFITS:
Rich in fiber, vitamins, and minerals, sweet potatoes promote general health.

NUTRITION PLAN: PER SERVING
Calories: 100, Protein: 2g, Carbohydrates: 24g, Fat: 0g

CUCUMBER TOMATO SALAD

COOKING TIME: 10 MINUTES, SERVING: MAKES 4 SERVINGS

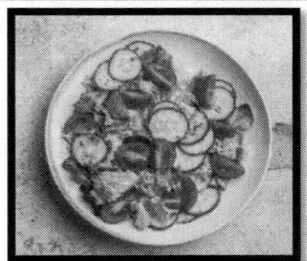

This crisp salad of tomatoes and cucumbers with vinegar, olive oil, and herbs is a cost-effective side dish.

INGREDIENTS:
- ☐ Two cucumbers, sliced
- ☐ Two tomatoes, diced
- ☐ 2 tbsp olive oil
- ☐ 1 tbsp vinegar
- ☐ 1 tsp dried herbs (basil, oregano)
- ☐ Salt and pepper to taste

STEP-BY-STEP INSTRUCTIONS:
1. Put the tomatoes and cucumbers in a basin.
2. Toss to coat after drizzling with vinegar and olive oil.
3. Add pepper, salt, and herbs for seasoning.

BENEFITS:
This salad is a perfect complement to any meal because it is high in vitamins and low in calories.

NUTRITION PLAN: PER SERVING
Calories: 70, Protein: 1g, Carbohydrates: 8g, Fat: 5g

MEAL PLAN CHARTS FOR 30 DAYS

This is a 30-day meal plan that includes inexpensive dishes from Dr. Nowzaradan's Meal Plan on a Budget. The total amount of calories consumed in a day stays below 1200 calories according to Dr. Nowzaradan's recommendations:

S/N	TIME	RECIPES
01	BREAKFAST	Oatmeal with Banana Slices
	LUNCH	Chickpea Salad
	DINNER	Spaghetti Aglio e Olio
	SNACK	Popcorn, Greek Yogurt with Berries
	SIDE DISH	Roasted Vegetables
02	BREAKFAST	Egg Muffins
	LUNCH	Veggie Wrap
	DINNER	Baked Chicken Drumsticks
	SNACK	Carrot Sticks with Hummus, Cottage Cheese with Pineapple
	SIDE DISH	Quinoa Pilaf
03	BREAKFAST	Peanut Butter Banana Toast
	LUNCH	Tuna Salad Sandwich
	DINNER	Veggie Stir-Fry with Tofu
	SNACK	Rice Cakes with Almond Butter, Hard-Boiled Eggs
	SIDE DISH	Black Bean Salad
04	BREAKFAST	Yogurt with Granola
	LUNCH	Black Bean Quesadillas
	DINNER	One-Pot Chili
	SNACK	Trail Mix, Greek Yogurt with Berries
	SIDE DISH	Steamed Broccoli
05	BREAKFAST	Breakfast Quesadilla
	LUNCH	Lentil Soup
	DINNER	Stuffed Bell Peppers with Rice and Beans
	SNACK	Celery Sticks with Peanut Butter, Cottage Cheese with Pineapple
	SIDE DISH	Rice and Beans
06	BREAKFAST	Banana Pancakes
	LUNCH	Quinoa Salad with Veggies
	DINNER	Baked Fish Fillets
	SNACK	Hard-boiled eggs, Greek Yogurt with Berries
	SIDE DISH	Mashed Sweet Potatoes
07	BREAKFAST	Breakfast Burrito Bowl
	LUNCH	Rice and Bean Bowl
	DINNER	Veggie Pasta Bake
	SNACK	Popcorn, Carrot Sticks with Hummus
	SIDE DISH	Cucumber Tomato Salad
08	BREAKFAST	Avocado Toast with Hard-Boiled Egg
	LUNCH	Pasta Primavera
	DINNER	Bean and Vegetable Casserole
	SNACK	Rice Cakes with Almond Butter, Greek Yogurt with Berries
	SIDE DISH	Black Bean Salad
09	BREAKFAST	Oatmeal with Banana Slices
	LUNCH	Chickpea Salad
	DINNER	Veggie Stir-Fry with Tofu
	SNACK	Trail Mix, Hard-Boiled Eggs
	SIDE DISH	Roasted Vegetables
10	BREAKFAST	Peanut Butter Banana Toast
	LUNCH	Tuna Salad Sandwich
	DINNER	Stuffed Bell Peppers with Rice and Beans
	SNACK	Popcorn, Greek Yogurt with Berries
	SIDE DISH	Steamed Broccoli

11	BREAKFAST	Yogurt with Granola
	LUNCH	Black Bean Quesadillas
	DINNER	Baked Chicken Drumsticks
	SNACK	Carrot Sticks with Hummus, Cottage Cheese with Pineapple
	SIDE DISH	Quinoa Pilaf
12	BREAKFAST	Breakfast Quesadilla
	LUNCH	Lentil Soup
	DINNER	Spaghetti Aglio e Olio
	SNACK	Rice Cakes with Almond Butter, Greek Yogurt with Berries
	SIDE DISH	Mashed Sweet Potatoes
13	BREAKFAST	Banana Pancakes
	LUNCH	Quinoa Salad with Veggies
	DINNER	Veggie Pasta Bake
	SNACK	Trail Mix, Hard-Boiled Eggs
	SIDE DISH	Cucumber Tomato Salad
14	BREAKFAST	Breakfast Burrito Bowl
	LUNCH	Rice and Bean Bowl
	DINNER	One-Pot Chili
	SNACK	Popcorn, Carrot Sticks with Hummus
	SIDE DISH	Rice and Beans
15	BREAKFAST	Egg Muffins
	LUNCH	Veggie Wrap
	DINNER	Baked Fish Fillets
	SNACK	Rice Cakes with Almond Butter, Greek Yogurt with Berries
	SIDE DISH	Black Bean Salad
16	BREAKFAST	Peanut Butter Banana Toast
	LUNCH	Tuna Salad Sandwich
	DINNER	Veggie Stir-Fry with Tofu
	SNACK	Popcorn, Carrot Sticks with Hummus
	SIDE DISH	Steamed Broccoli
17	BREAKFAST	Yogurt with Granola
	LUNCH	Black Bean Quesadillas
	DINNER	Bean and Vegetable Casserole
	SNACK	Trail Mix, Greek Yogurt with Berries
	SIDE DISH	Quinoa Pilaf
18	BREAKFAST	Oatmeal with Banana Slices
	LUNCH	Chickpea Salad
	DINNER	Stuffed Bell Peppers with Rice and Beans
	SNACK	Rice Cakes with Almond Butter, Cottage Cheese with Pineapple
	SIDE DISH	Roasted Vegetables
19	BREAKFAST	Breakfast Quesadilla
	LUNCH	Lentil Soup
	DINNER	Spaghetti Aglio e Olio
	SNACK	Hard-boiled eggs, Greek Yogurt with Berries
	SIDE DISH	Mashed Sweet Potatoes
20	BREAKFAST	Banana Pancakes
	LUNCH	Quinoa Salad with Veggies
	DINNER	Veggie Pasta Bake
	SNACK	Popcorn, Carrot Sticks with Hummus
	SIDE DISH	Cucumber Tomato Salad
21	BREAKFAST	Breakfast Burrito Bowl
	LUNCH	Rice and Bean Bowl
	DINNER	One-Pot Chili

	SNACK	Trail Mix, Greek Yogurt with Berries
	SIDE DISH	Rice and Beans
22	BREAKFAST	Avocado Toast with Hard-Boiled Egg
	LUNCH	Pasta Primavera
	DINNER	Baked Chicken Drumsticks
	SNACK	Rice Cakes with Almond Butter, Greek Yogurt with Berries
	SIDE DISH	Black Bean Salad
23	BREAKFAST	Oatmeal with Banana Slices
	LUNCH	Chickpea Salad
	DINNER	Veggie Stir-Fry with Tofu
	SNACK	Popcorn, Carrot Sticks with Hummus
	SIDE DISH	Steamed Broccoli
24	BREAKFAST	Peanut Butter Banana Toast
	LUNCH	Tuna Salad Sandwich
	DINNER	Stuffed Bell Peppers with Rice and Beans
	SNACK	Trail Mix, Greek Yogurt with Berries
	SIDE DISH	Quinoa Pilaf
25	BREAKFAST	Yogurt with Granola
	LUNCH	Black Bean Quesadillas
	DINNER	Bean and Vegetable Casserole
	SNACK	Rice Cakes with Almond Butter, Cottage Cheese with Pineapple
	SIDE DISH	Roasted Vegetables
26	BREAKFAST	Breakfast Quesadilla
	LUNCH	Lentil Soup
	DINNER	Spaghetti Aglio e Olio
	SNACK	Hard-boiled eggs, Greek Yogurt with Berries
	SIDE DISH	Mashed Sweet Potatoes
27	BREAKFAST	Banana Pancakes
	LUNCH	Quinoa Salad with Veggies
	DINNER	Veggie Pasta Bake
	SNACK	Popcorn, Carrot Sticks with Hummus
	SIDE DISH	Cucumber Tomato Salad
28	BREAKFAST	Breakfast Burrito Bowl
	LUNCH	Rice and Bean Bowl
	DINNER	One-Pot Chili
	SNACK	Trail Mix, Greek Yogurt with Berries
	SIDE DISH	Rice and Beans
29	BREAKFAST	Egg Muffins
	LUNCH	Veggie Wrap
	DINNER	Baked Fish Fillets
	SNACK	Rice Cakes with Almond Butter, Greek Yogurt with Berries
	SIDE DISH	Black Bean Salad
30	BREAKFAST	Peanut Butter Banana Toast
	LUNCH	Tuna Salad Sandwich
	DINNER	Veggie Stir-Fry with Tofu
	SNACK	Popcorn, Carrot Sticks with Hummus
	SIDE DISH	Steamed Broccoli

DR. NOWZARADAN'S LOW CARB HIGH PROTEIN RECIPES

Welcome to Dr. Nowzaradan's low-carb/High-Protein Recipes! As Dr. Nowzaradan advocates, we'll look at delicious and nutritious recipes that are low in carbs and high in protein. These recipes are intended to help you reach your health and weight loss objectives while providing enjoyable and flavorful meals. Let's explore the world of low-carb, high-protein cookery with Dr. Nowzaradan's help.

INTRODUCTION

Low-carb, high-protein diets have become increasingly popular in the health and nutrition fields because they may help with weight loss, enhance metabolic health, and boost satiety. Renowned bariatric surgeon Dr. Nowzaradan understands how crucial it is to include these ideas in diet regimens for people who want to lose weight and get healthier overall.

We'll discuss Dr. Nowzaradan's low-carb, high-protein dietary philosophy while highlighting tasty and filling foods that follow his advice. These recipes will provide wholesome options to help you on your journey, whether you want to lose weight, control your blood sugar, or live a healthy lifestyle.

Every recipe, from filling main courses to tasty snacks and sides, is designed to be both tasty and nourishing, assisting you in sticking to your wellness and health objectives. You may take significant strides toward a healthier, happier self by including these recipes in your meal planning and adhering to Dr. Nowzaradan's advice.

BREAKFAST RECIPES

SPINACH AND FETA OMELETTE

COOKING TIME: 10 MINUTES, SERVING: MAKES 1 SERVING

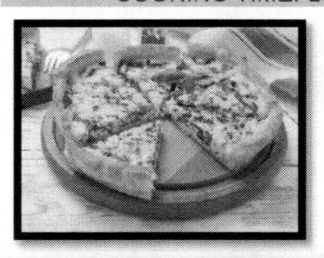

A fluffy omelet filled with nutrient-rich spinach and creamy feta cheese.

INGREDIENTS:
- Two eggs
- 1/2 cup fresh spinach, chopped
- 1/4 cup feta cheese, crumbled
- 1 tsp olive oil
- Salt and pepper to taste

STEP-BY-STEP INSTRUCTIONS:
1. Add the eggs, salt, and pepper to a bowl and whisk.
2. In a non-stick skillet set over medium heat, warm the olive oil.
3. After adding, boil the spinach until it wilts.
4. When the eggs are almost set, pour them over the spinach.
5. One-half of the omelet should have feta cheese on it.
6. Fold the omelet in half once the cheese has melted and continue cooking for another minute.

BENEFITS:
The spinach provides a lot of vitamins and protein to this omelet.

NUTRITION PLAN: PER SERVING
Calories: 220, Protein: 14g, Carbohydrates: 2g, Fat: 18g

CRUSTLESS QUICHE WITH BACON AND CHEDDAR

COOKING TIME: 40 MINUTES, SERVING: MAKES 6 SERVINGS

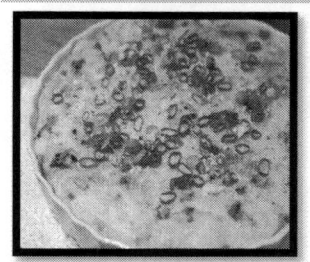

It is a tasty quiche without the hefty carbs, a total of sharp cheddar cheese and flavorful bacon.

INGREDIENTS:
- Six eggs
- 1 cup cheddar cheese, shredded
- Four slices of bacon, cooked and crumbled
- 1 cup milk (dairy or non-dairy)
- 1/2 cup chopped green onions
- Salt and pepper to taste

STEP-BY-STEP INSTRUCTIONS:
1. Set the oven's temperature to 175°C/350°F.
2. Whisk the eggs, milk, pepper, and salt in a bowl.
3. Add the green onions, bacon, and cheddar cheese and stir.
4. Transfer mixture to pie dish that has been oiled.
5. Bake for 30 to 35 minutes or until golden brown and firm.

BENEFITS:
This quiche has a high protein,, healthy fat, and low carb content.

NUTRITION PLAN: PER SERVING
Calories: 250, Protein: 15g, Carbohydrates: 4g, Fat: 20g

GREEK YOGURT PARFAIT WITH BERRIES AND ALMONDS

COOKING TIME: 5 MINUTES, SERVING: MAKES 1 SERVING

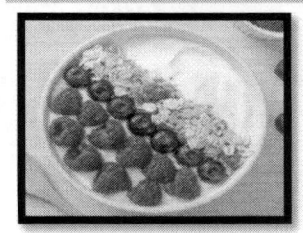

Protein-rich breakfast treat of creamy Greek yogurt mixed with crunchy almonds and juicy berries.

INGREDIENTS:
- 1 cup Greek yogurt
- 1/2 cup mixed berries (strawberries, blueberries, raspberries)
- 2 tbsp sliced almonds
- 1 tsp honey (optional)

STEP-BY-STEP INSTRUCTIONS:
1. Arrange half of the yogurt, then half of the berries and almonds in a bowl or glass.
2. Repeat the layering process with the remaining yogurt, berries, and almonds.
3. If desired, drizzle with honey.

BENEFITS:
This parfait is high in antioxidants, healthy fats, and protein.

NUTRITION PLAN: PER SERVING
Calories: 200, Protein: 15g, Carbohydrates: 20g, Fat: 8g

VEGGIE BREAKFAST CASSEROLE

COOKING TIME: 45 MINUTES, SERVING: MAKES 6 SERVINGS

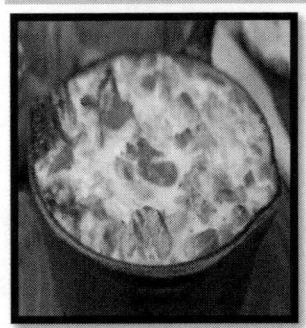

A filling breakfast dish consisting of lean turkey sausage, diced veggies, and eggs in a substantial casserole.

INGREDIENTS:
- Eight eggs
- 1 cup diced bell peppers
- 1 cup diced zucchini
- 1 cup chopped spinach
- 1/2 lb lean turkey sausage, cooked and crumbled
- 1 cup shredded cheese (optional)
- Salt and pepper to taste

STEP-BY-STEP INSTRUCTIONS:
1. Set oven temperature to 350°F (175°C).
2. Mix the eggs, pepper, and salt in a big basin.
3. Add the turkey sausage, bell peppers, zucchini, spinach, and cheese, and stir.
4. Spoon the mixture into a baking dish that has been buttered.
5. Bake until firm and golden brown, 35 to 40 minutes.

BENIFITS:
This casserole has a lot of protein and veggies for extra nutrition.

NUTRITION PLAN: PER SERVING
Calories: 230, Protein: 20g, Carbohydrates: 5g, Fat: 15g

LOW-CARB PROTEIN PANCAKES

COOKING TIME: 15 MINUTES, SERVING: MAKES 2 SERVINGS

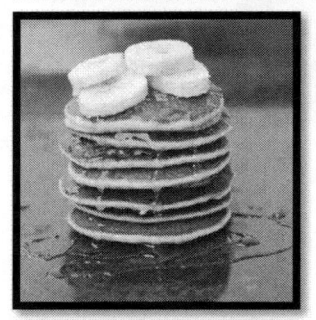

Made with protein powder and almond flour, these fluffy pancakes are garnished with sliced strawberries and a dollop of Greek yogurt.

INGREDIENTS:
- 1/2 cup almond flour
- One scoop of protein powder
- Two eggs
- 1/4 cup milk (dairy or non-dairy)
- 1 tsp baking powder
- 1/2 cup sliced strawberries
- 1/4 cup Greek yogurt

STEP-BY-STEP INSTRUCTIONS:
1. Combine the protein powder, baking powder, and almond flour in a bowl.
2. Beat the eggs and milk together in a separate bowl.
3. Smoothly blend the dry and wet components.
4. Pour the mixture into a non-stick skillet set over medium heat to form little pancakes.
5. Cook until surface bubbles appear, then turn and cook until golden brown.
6. Top with cut strawberries and Greek yogurt, and serve.

BENEFITS:

These pancakes are ideal for a healthy meal because they are high in protein and low in carbohydrates.

NUTRITION PLAN: PER SERVING
Calories: 250, Protein: 20g, Carbohydrates: 10g, Fat: 15g

SMOKED SALMON AND AVOCADO TOAST

COOKING TIME: 5 MINUTES, SERVING: MAKES 1 SERVING

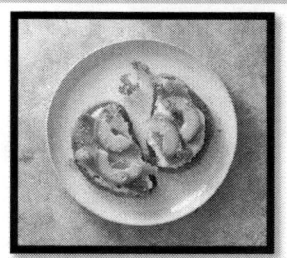

A posh and high-protein breakfast choice is whole-grain bread with smoked salmon and creamy avocado slices on top.

INGREDIENTS:
- One slice whole grain bread
- 1/2 avocado, mashed
- 2 oz smoked salmon
- 1 tsp lemon juice
- Salt and pepper to taste

STEP-BY-STEP INSTRUCTIONS:
1. Toast the bread with whole grains.
2. Add the lemon juice, salt, and pepper, and mash the avocado.
3. On the bread, distribute the avocado.
4. Add smoked salmon on top.

BENEFITS:
Omega-3 fatty acids, protein, and good fats abound in this breakfast.

NUTRITION PLAN: PER SERVING
Calories: 300, Protein: 15g, Carbohydrates: 20g, Fat: 20g

COTTAGE CHEESE AND BERRY BOWL

COOKING TIME: 5 MINUTES, SERVING: MAKES 1 SERVING

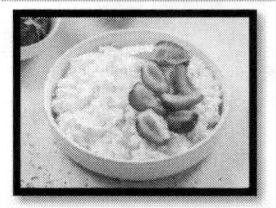

Sweet berries, a honey drizzle, and creamy cottage cheese make for a leisurely but filling breakfast.

INGREDIENTS:
- 1 cup cottage cheese
- 1/2 cup mixed berries (strawberries, blueberries, raspberries)
- 1 tsp honey (optional)

STEP-BY-STEP INSTRUCTIONS:
1. The cottage cheese should be put in a bowl.
2. Add a mixture of berries on top.
3. If desired, drizzle with honey.

BENEFITS:
This bowl has a decent macronutrient balance and is heavy in protein.

NUTRITION PLAN: PER SERVING
Calories: 200, Protein: 15g, Carbohydrates: 15g, Fat: 5g

EGG AND VEGGIE MUFFIN CUPS
COOKING TIME: 25 MINUTES, SERVING: MAKES 6 SERVINGS

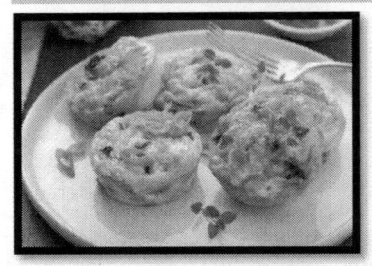

These portable muffin cups are stuffed with scrambled eggs, sliced veggies, and shredded cheese, perfect for an on-the-go breakfast choice.

INGREDIENTS:
- Six eggs
- 1 cup diced vegetables (bell peppers, onions, spinach)
- 1/2 cup shredded cheese
- Salt and pepper to taste

STEP-BY-STEP INSTRUCTIONS:
1. Preheat the oven to 350°F (175°C).
2. In a bowl, whisk the egg with salt and pepper.
3. Stir in the diced vegetables and shredded cheese.
4. Pour the mixture into a greased muffin tin, filling each cup about three-quarters full.
5. Bake for 20-25 minutes, until the eggs are set and lightly browned on top.

BENEFITS:
These muffin cups are high in protein and convenient for meal prepping or on-the-go breakfasts.

NUTRITION PLAN: PER MUFFIN CUP
Calories: 100, Protein: 7, Carbohydrates: 2g, Fat: 7g

LUNCH RECIPES

GRILLED CHICKEN CAESAR SALAD
COOKING TIME: 20 MINUTES, SERVING: 2 SERVINGS

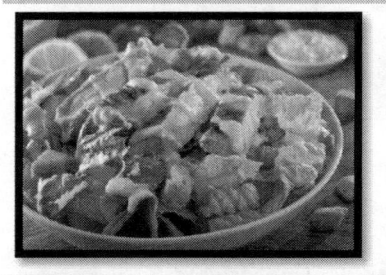

A traditional Caesar salad with extra protein from grilled chicken.

INGREDIENTS:
- Two chicken breasts
- 4 cups romaine lettuce, chopped
- 1/4 cup shaved Parmesan cheese
- Two tablespoons Caesar dressing (low-fat)
- Salt and pepper to taste

STEP-BY-STEP INSTRUCTIONS:
1. Add salt and pepper to chicken breasts for seasoning.
2. The chicken breasts should be cooked through after 6 to 8 minutes on each side of the grill over medium heat.
3. After a few minutes of resting, slice the chicken.
4. Combine the romaine lettuce and Caesar dressing in a big bowl.
5. Add shaved Parmesan cheese and sliced grilled chicken on top.

BENEFITS:
Low in carbohydrates and high in protein.

NUTRITION PLAN: PER SERVING

Calories: 300, Protein: 35g, Carbohydrates: 8g, Fat: 15g

TURKEY AND AVOCADO WRAP
COOKING TIME: 10 MINUTES, SERVING: 1 SERVING

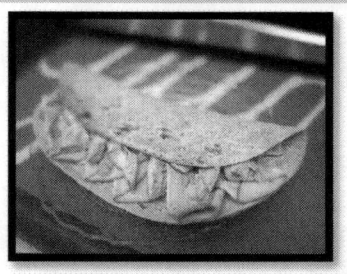

It is a simple yet filling wrap high in healthy fats and lean turkey.

INGREDIENTS:
- One whole-grain wrap
- Four slices of turkey breast
- 1/2 avocado, sliced
- 1/2 cup lettuce
- One tomato, sliced
- Salt and pepper to taste

STEP-BY-STEP INSTRUCTIONS:
1. Transfer the wrap to a level surface.
2. Arrange the turkey breast, avocado slices, tomato, lettuce, and wrap in layers.
3. Add pepper and salt for seasoning.
4. After tightly rolling the wrap, cut it in half.

BENEFITS:
Offers a healthy balance of fats and proteins.

NUTRITION PLAN: PER SERVING
Calories: 350, Protein: 25g, Carbohydrates: 30g, Fat: 15g

TUNA SALAD LETTUCE WRAPS
COOKING TIME: 15 MINUTES, SERVING: 2 SERVINGS

A light and refreshing lunch option.

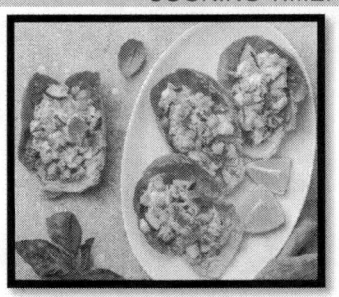

INGREDIENTS:
- One can of tuna in water, drained
- 1/4 cup Greek yogurt
- One celery stalk, diced
- One tablespoon of fresh herbs (parsley, dill, etc.), chopped
- One tablespoon of lemon juice
- Salt and pepper to taste
- Four large lettuce leaves

STEP-BY-STEP INSTRUCTIONS:
1. Combine the tuna, Greek yogurt, celery, herbs, lemon juice, salt, and pepper in a bowl.
2. Fill lettuce leaves with the tuna salad.
3. The lettuce leaves can be rolled or folded to envelop the filling.

BENEFITS:
Low in carbohydrates and high in protein.

NUTRITION PLAN: PER SERVING
Calories: 200, Protein: 25g, Carbohydrates: 5g, Fat: 8g

ZUCCHINI NOODLE STIR-FRY WITH CHICKEN

COOKING TIME: 20 MINUTES, SERVING: 2 SERVINGS

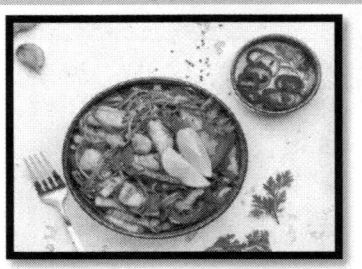

A low-carb take on the classic stir-fry.

INGREDIENTS:
- Two chicken breasts, thinly sliced
- Two medium zucchinis, spiralized
- One bell pepper, sliced
- 1 cup broccoli florets
- Two tablespoons soy sauce (low-sodium)
- One tablespoon of olive oil
- One clove of garlic, minced

STEP-BY-STEP INSTRUCTIONS:
1. In a big skillet, warm up the olive oil over medium-high heat.
2. Add the chicken slices and simmer for about 5 minutes until browned.
3. For three to four minutes, stir-fry the broccoli, bell pepper, and garlic.
4. After adding the zucchini noodles and soy sauce, cook for two to three minutes or until everything is heated.

BENEFITS:
High in protein and fiber and low in carbohydrates.

NUTRITION PLAN: PER SERVING
Calories: 250, Protein: 30g, Carbohydrates: 12g, Fat: 10g

EGG SALAD STUFFED BELL PEPPERS

COOKING TIME: 15 MINUTES, SERVING: 2 SERVINGS

A unique way to consume egg salad.

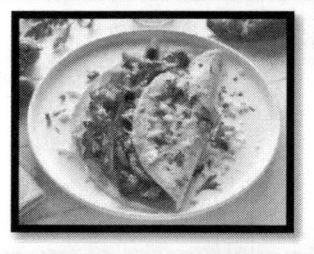

INGREDIENTS:
- Four hard-boiled eggs, chopped
- 1/4 cup Greek yogurt
- One tablespoon of Dijon mustard
- One celery stalk, diced
- Salt and pepper to taste
- Two bell peppers, halved and seeded

STEP-BY-STEP INSTRUCTIONS:
1. Combine chopped eggs, Greek yogurt, celery, mustard, and salt & pepper in a bowl.
2. Fill the split bell peppers with the egg salad using a spoon.

BENEFITS:
Low in carbohydrates and high in protein.

NUTRITION PLAN: PER SERVING
Calories: 200, Protein: 15g, Carbohydrates: 10g, Fat: 10g

SHRIMP AND VEGGIE SKEWERS

COOKING TIME: 20 MINUTES, SERVING: 2 SERVINGS

Delicious and light grilled skewers.

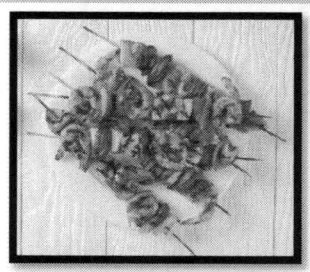

INGREDIENTS:
- [ ] 12 large shrimp, peeled and deveined
- [ ] 1 cup cherry tomatoes
- [ ] One zucchini, sliced
- [ ] One bell pepper, cut into chunks
- [ ] Two tablespoons of olive oil
- [ ] One tablespoon of lemon juice
- [ ] Salt and pepper to taste

STEP-BY-STEP INSTRUCTIONS:
1. Grill at a medium-high temperature.
2. In a bowl, combine olive oil, lemon juice, salt, and pepper.
3. Put veggies and prawns on skewers.
4. Apply a layer of the olive oil mixture.
5. Until the vegetables are soft and the shrimp are opaque, grill for 3–4 minutes on each side.

BENEFITS:
Low in calories and high in protein.

NUTRITION PLAN: PER SERVING
Calories: 220, Protein: 25g, Carbohydrates: 8g, Fat: 10g

CAULIFLOWER FRIED RICE WITH TOFU

COOKING TIME: 20 MINUTES, SERVING: 2 SERVINGS

A healthier take on fried rice.

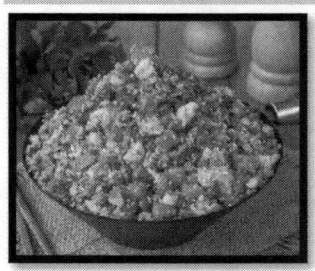

INGREDIENTS:
- [ ] One small head of cauliflower, riced
- [ ] 1 cup tofu, cubed
- [ ] 1/2 cup peas and carrots mix
- [ ] Two eggs scrambled
- [ ] Two tablespoons soy sauce (low-sodium)
- [ ] One tablespoon of sesame oil
- [ ] One clove of garlic, minced

STEP-BY-STEP INSTRUCTIONS:
1. Over medium-high heat, preheat the sesame oil in a large skillet.
2. For about five minutes, add the tofu and heat it until browned.
3. Cook for one more minute after adding the garlic.
4. For 3–4 minutes, stir-fry the riced cauliflower, peas, and carrots.
5. Remove from the skillet after pushing mixture to one side and scrambled eggs to the other; heat until eggs are set.
6. Blend everything after adding the soy sauce.

BENEFITS:
Abundant in plant-based protein and low in carbohydrates.

NUTRITION PLAN: PER SERVING

Calories: 250, Protein: 15g, Carbohydrates: 12g, Fat: 15g

GREEK CHICKEN SALAD BOWL

COOKING TIME: 20 MINUTES, SERVING: 2 SERVINGS

It's a light salad with a Mediterranean flair.

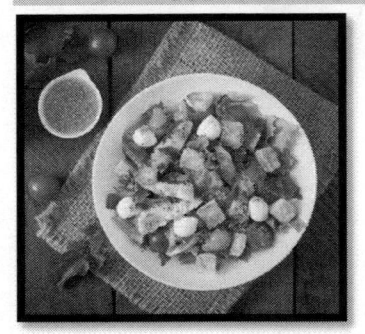

INGREDIENTS:
- Two chicken breasts, grilled and sliced
- One cucumber, diced
- 1 cup cherry tomatoes, halved
- 1/4 cup Kalamata olives, pitted
- 1/4 cup feta cheese, crumbled
- Two tablespoons of olive oil
- One tablespoon of lemon juice
- One teaspoon dried oregano
- Salt and pepper to taste

STEP-BY-STEP INSTRUCTIONS:
1. Combine cucumber, olives, cherry tomatoes, and feta cheese in a big bowl.
2. Mix the olive oil, lemon juice, oregano, salt, and pepper in a small bowl.
3. Pour the dressing over everything in the big bowl, add the grilled chicken, and stir to mix.

BENEFITS:
Rich in fiber, healthy fats, and high protein.

NUTRITION PLAN: PER SERVING
Calories: 350 per serving, Protein: 30g, Carbohydrates: 10g, Fat: 20g

DINNER RECIPES

BAKED SALMON WITH ASPARAGUS

COOKING TIME: 25 MINUTES, SERVING: 2 SERVINGS

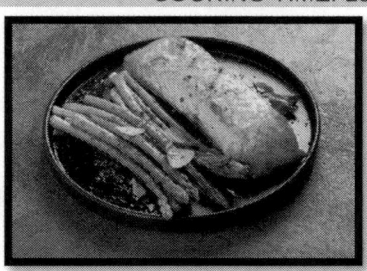

Warm salmon fillets cooked with herbs and lemon and spears of roasted asparagus.

INGREDIENTS:
- Two salmon fillets
- One bunch of asparagus, trimmed
- One lemon, sliced
- Two tablespoons of olive oil
- One teaspoon of dried dill
- Salt and pepper to taste

STEP-BY-STEP INSTRUCTIONS:
1. Set oven temperature to 400°F or 200°C.
2. Arrange the asparagus and salmon fillets on a baking sheet.
3. Add a drizzle of olive oil and season with salt, pepper, and dill.
4. Place slivers of lemon over the fish.
5. Bake for 15 to 20 minutes until the asparagus is soft and the salmon is cooked.

BENEFITS:

Low in carbohydrates, high in protein and omega-3 fatty acids.

NUTRITION PLAN: PER SERVING
Calories: 350, Protein: 35g, Carbohydrates: 5g, Fat: 20g

TURKEY MEATBALLS WITH ZOODLES

COOKING TIME: 30 MINUTES, SERVING: 2 SERVINGS

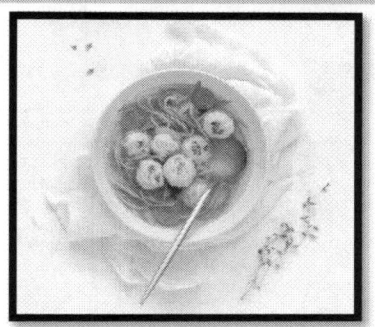

Spiralized zucchini noodles and marinara sauce accompany homemade turkey meatballs.

INGREDIENTS:
- 1 lb ground turkey
- 1/4 cup breadcrumbs
- One egg
- One teaspoon of Italian seasoning
- Two zucchinis, spiralized
- 1 cup marinara sauce
- One tablespoon of olive oil
- Salt and pepper to taste

STEP-BY-STEP INSTRUCTIONS:
1. Turn the oven on to 375°F, or 190°C.
2. Combine the ground turkey, breadcrumbs, egg, salt, pepper, and Italian seasoning in a bowl. Shape into meatballs.
3. Meatballs should be baked on a baking sheet for 15 to 20 minutes or until done.
4. In a skillet with heated olive oil, sauté the zucchini for two to three minutes.
5. Serve the warm marinara sauce with meatballs on top of zoodles.

BENEFITS:
Abundant in vegetables, high in protein, and low in carbohydrates.

NUTRITION PLAN: PER SERVING
Calories: 300, Protein: 30g, Carbohydrates: 12g, Fat: 15g

SPAGHETTI SQUASH WITH CHICKEN ALFREDO

COOKING TIME: 45 MINUTES, SERVING: 2 SERVINGS

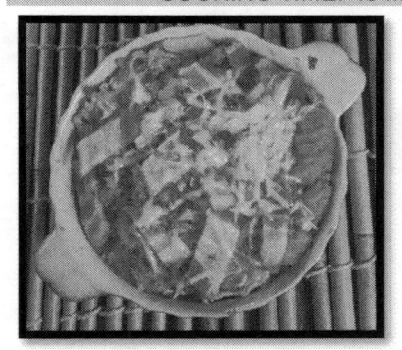

Greek yogurt and Parmesan cheese are combined to make a creamy Alfredo sauce served with roasted spaghetti squash and grilled chicken breast.

INGREDIENTS:
- One medium spaghetti squash
- Two chicken breasts
- 1 cup Greek yogurt
- 1/2 cup grated Parmesan cheese
- Two cloves garlic, minced
- One tablespoon of olive oil
- Salt and pepper to taste

STEP-BY-STEP INSTRUCTIONS:
1. Turn the oven on to 400°F or 200°C. Scoop out the seeds, split the spaghetti squash in half, and roast it cut-side down for 30 to 40 minutes until it gets soft.

2. Chicken breasts should be seasoned with salt and pepper, grilled until done, and then sliced.
3. Garlic should be fragrantly sautéed in hot olive oil in a pan. Stir in the Parmesan cheese and Greek yogurt until smooth.
4. Scrape out spaghetti squash threads with a fork and combine with sliced chicken and Alfredo sauce.

BENEFITS:
Creamy, delicious texture; high in protein and low in carbohydrates.

NUTRITION PLAN: PER SERVING
Calories: 400, Protein: 35g, Carbohydrates: 15g, Fat: 20g

BEEF AND BROCCOLI STIR-FRY

COOKING TIME: 25 MINUTES, SERVING: 2 SERVINGS

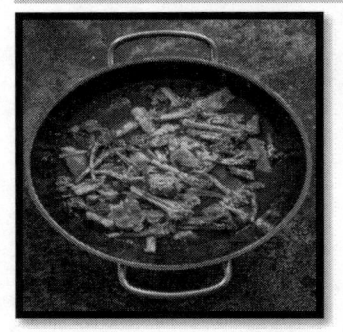

Stir-fried, thinly sliced beef with onions, bell peppers, and broccoli florets in a flavorful ginger-soy sauce.

INGREDIENTS:
- 1/2 lb beef sirloin, thinly sliced
- 2 cups broccoli florets
- One bell pepper, sliced
- 1/2 onion, sliced
- Two tablespoons soy sauce (low-sodium)
- One tablespoon of olive oil
- One tablespoon grated ginger
- Two cloves garlic, minced

STEP-BY-STEP INSTRUCTIONS:
1. Warm the olive oil over medium-high heat in a big skillet or wok.
2. Add the steak and heat for 3–4 minutes until browned.
3. Stir-fry the onion, bell pepper, ginger, and garlic for two to three minutes.
4. Add the broccoli and soy sauce, and cook for about 5 minutes or until the broccoli is soft.

BENEFITS:
Low in carbohydra.tes and high in protein and fiber.

NUTRITION PLAN: PER SERVING
Calories: 350, Protein: 30g, Carbohydrates: 10g, Fat: 20g

STUFFED PORTOBELLO MUSHROOMS

COOKING TIME: 30 MINUTES, SERVING: 2 SERVINGS

Caps are baked till golden and bubbling.

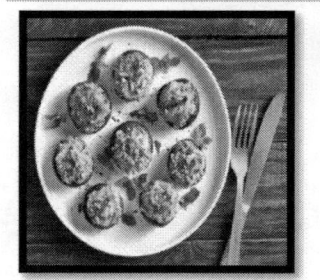

INGREDIENTS:
- Four large portobello mushroom caps
- 1/2 lb ground turkey
- 1 cup spinach, chopped
- 1/2 cup shredded mozzarella cheese
- One tablespoon of olive oil
- One clove of garlic, minced
- Salt and pepper to taste

STEP-BY-STEP INSTRUCTIONS:
1. Turn the oven on to 375°F, or 190°C.
2. After removing the mushroom stems, oil the caps with olive oil.
3. Cook the ground turkey and garlic in a skillet until browned. When the spinach begins to wilt, add it.
4. Place the turkey mixture inside the mushrooms and cover with mozzarella cheese.
5. Bake for 15 to 20 minutes until the cheese is melted and the mushrooms are soft.

BENEFITS:
Rich in veggies and protein, low in carbohydrates.

NUTRITION PLAN: PER SERVING
Calories: 300, Protein: 25g, Carbohydrates: 10g, Fat: 15g

GRILLED LEMON HERB CHICKEN

COOKING TIME: 30 MINUTES, SERVING: 2 SERVINGS

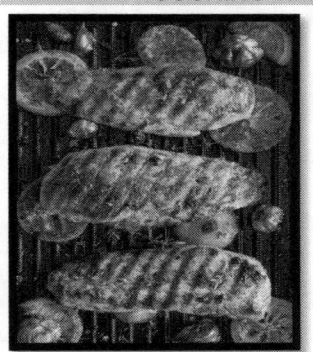

Serve succulent chicken breasts with a side order of steamed green beans, marinated in a zesty lemon-herb sauce and cooked to perfection on the grill.

INGREDIENTS:
- ☐ Two chicken breasts
- ☐ One lemon, juiced
- ☐ Two tablespoons of olive oil
- ☐ One teaspoon dried oregano
- ☐ One teaspoon of dried thyme
- ☐ One garlic clove, minced
- ☐ Salt and pepper to taste
- ☐ 1 cup green beans, steamed

STEP-BY-STEP INSTRUCTIONS:
1. In a bowl, combine the lemon juice, olive oil, garlic, thyme, oregano, salt, and pepper.
2. Marinate the chicken breasts in the marinade for a minimum of fifteen minutes.
3. Grill at a medium-high temperature. Grill the chicken for 6–7 minutes on each side until cooked.
4. Alongside cooked green beans, serve.

BENEFITS:
Low in fat and carbohydrates and high in protein.

NUTRITION PLAN: PER SERVING
Calories: 280, Protein: 35g, Carbohydrates: 8g, Fat: 12g

CAULIFLOWER CRUST PIZZA
COOKING TIME: 40 MINUTES, SERVING: 2 SERVINGS

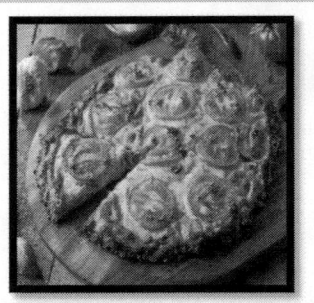

A handcrafted pizza dough made with shredded cheese, marinara sauce, and your preferred pizza toppings.

INGREDIENTS:
- One small head of cauliflower, riced
- One egg, beaten
- 1 cup shredded mozzarella cheese
- 1/4 cup grated Parmesan cheese
- 1 cup marinara sauce
- 1 cup desired toppings
- Salt and pepper to taste

STEP-BY-STEP INSTRUCTIONS:
1. Aim for 425°F (220°C) in the oven.
2. After 5–6 minutes in the microwave, rice the cauliflower and press out any extra moisture.
3. Combine the cauliflower, egg, Parmesan, mozzarella, and salt and pepper in a bowl.
4. Press the mixture onto a baking sheet lined with parchment paper to form a crust.
5. Coat in the oven for 15 to 20 minutes till browned.
6. Add cheese, marinara sauce, and other preferred toppings on top. Bake for an additional ten minutes.

BENEFITS:
Rich in vegetables and protein, low in carbohydrates.

NUTRITION PLAN: PER SERVING
Calories: 300, Protein: 20g, Carbohydrates: 15g, Fat: 20g

BAKED COD WITH TOMATO BASIL RELISH
COOKING TIME: 25 MINUTES, SERVING: 2 SERVINGS

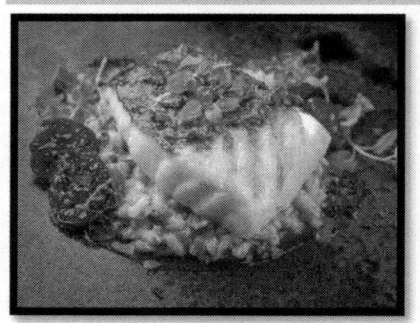

Lightly seasoned cod fillets baked with fresh tomatoes and basil relish, accompanied by sautéed spinach on the side.

INGREDIENTS:
- Two cod fillets
- Two tomatoes, diced
- 1/4 cup fresh basil, chopped
- One tablespoon of olive oil
- One clove of garlic, minced
- Salt and pepper to taste
- 2 cups spinach, sautéed

STEP-BY-STEP INSTRUCTIONS:
1. Turn the oven on to 400°F or 200°C.
2. Cod fillets should be seasoned with salt and pepper and placed on a baking sheet.
3. Combine tomatoes, basil, garlic, olive oil, salt, and pepper in a bowl. Place a spoon over the cod.
4. Bake until the cod is thoroughly done, 15 to 20 minutes.
5. Garlic and a small amount of olive oil are used to sauté spinach.

6. Serve sautéed spinach alongside cod.

BENEFITS:
Rich in protein and good fats, low in carbohydrates.

NUTRITION PLAN: PER SERVING
Calories: 250, Protein: 25g, Carbohydrates: 10g, Fat: 12g

SNACKS

GREEK YOGURT AND BERRY SMOOTHIE

COOKING TIME: 5 MINUTES, SERVING: 1 SERVING

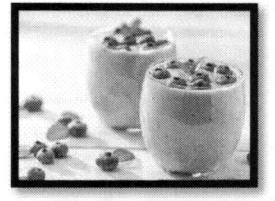

A delicious snack of creamy Greek yogurt, mixed berry smoothie with a dash of almond milk.

INGREDIENTS:
- 1 cup Greek yogurt
- 1 cup mixed berries (fresh or frozen)
- 1/2 cup unsweetened almond milk
- One tablespoon honey (optional)

STEP-BY-STEP INSTRUCTIONS:
1. Blend almond milk, Greek yogurt, and mixed berries in a blender.
2. Process till smooth.
3. If desired, add honey and mix one more.

BENEFITS:
Low in added sugars and high in protein and antioxidants.

NUTRITION PLAN: PER SERVING
Calories: 200, Protein: 15g, Carbohydrates: 25g, Fat: 5g

PROTEIN-PACKED DEVILED EGGS

COOKING TIME: 15 MINUTES, SERVING: 4 SERVINGS (8 HALVES)

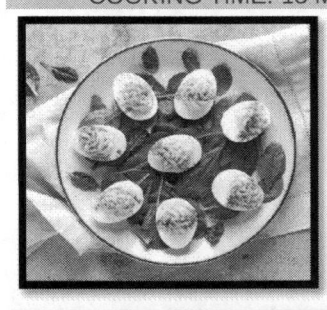

A snack high in protein can be made from hard-boiled eggs packed with a mixture of Greek yogurt, mustard, and minced herbs.

INGREDIENTS:
- Four hard-boiled eggs
- 1/4 cup Greek yogurt
- One teaspoon mustard
- One tablespoon of chopped fresh herbs (parsley, dill, etc.)
- Salt and pepper to taste

STEP-BY-STEP INSTRUCTIONS:
1. Take the hard-boiled eggs and cut them in half.
2. After removing the yolks, combine Greek yogurt, herbs, mustard, salt, and pepper.
3. Spoon the yolk mixture into the egg whites.

BENEFITS:
Rich in good fats and protein.

NUTRITION PLAN: PER HALF

Calories: 60, Protein: 5g, Carbohydrates: 1g, Fat: 4g

COTTAGE CHEESE AND TOMATO SLICES

COOKING TIME: 5 MINUTES, SERVING: 1 SERVING

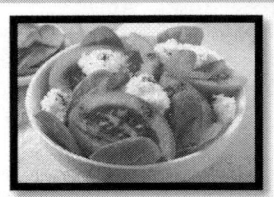

An easy and high-protein snack is creamy cottage cheese with sliced tomatoes and a dash of salt and pepper on top.

INGREDIENTS:
- 1 cup cottage cheese
- One medium tomato, sliced
- Salt and pepper to taste

STEP-BY-STEP INSTRUCTIONS:
1. Put cottage cheese into a dish.
2. Add slices of tomato on top.
3. Add pepper and salt for seasoning.

BENEFITS:
Rich in vitamins and protein.

NUTRITION PLAN: PER SERVING
Calories: 120, Protein: 14g, Carbohydrates: 6g, Fat: 5g

TURKEY AND CHEESE ROLL-UPS

COOKING TIME: 5 MINUTES, SERVING: 1 SERVING

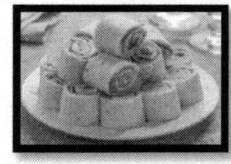

Rolling sliced turkey breast with a piece of cheese makes a quick and simple snack that is high in protein.

INGREDIENTS:
- Four slices of turkey breast
- Two slices cheese (cheddar, Swiss, etc.)

STEP-BY-STEP INSTRUCTIONS:
1. Top each piece of turkey with a slice of cheese.
2. If necessary, roll up and fasten with a toothpick.

BENEFITS:
Low in carbohydrates and high in protein.

NUTRITION PLAN: PER SERVING
Calories: 150, Protein: 18g, Carbohydrates: 2g, Fat: 8g

ROASTED CHICKPEAS

COOKING TIME: 30 MINUTES, SERVING: 2 SERVINGS

Crunchy and filling snack of crispy roasted chickpeas seasoned.

INGREDIENTS:
- One can of chickpeas, drained and rinsed
- One tablespoon of olive oil
- One teaspoon of paprika (or your favorite spice blend)
- Salt to taste

STEP-BY-STEP INSTRUCTIONS:
1. Turn the oven on to 400°F or 200°C.
2. Add salt, paprika, and olive oil to the chickpeas.
3. Place on a baking sheet, then roast until crispy, 20 to 30 minutes.

BENEFITS:
Rich in protein and fiber.

NUTRITION PLAN: PER SERVING
Calories: 200, Protein: 10g, Carbohydrates: 30g, Fat: 8g

CHEESE AND VEGGIE PLATTER

COOKING TIME: 10 MINUTES, SERVING: 2 SERVINGS

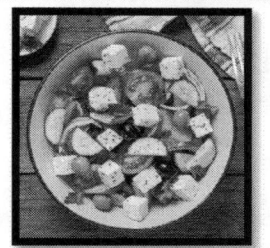

Various sliced cheese, cucumber, cherry tomatoes, and bell peppers make a nourishing and adaptable snack.

INGREDIENTS:
- Four slices cheese (cheddar, mozzarella, etc.)
- One cucumber, sliced
- One bell pepper, sliced
- 1 cup cherry tomatoes

STEP-BY-STEP INSTRUCTIONS:
1. Put the cheese and the cut veggies on a serving dish.

BENEFITS:
A well-balanced combination of fiber, protein, and good fats.

NUTRITION PLAN: PER SERVING
Calories: 200, Protein: 10g, Carbohydrates: 15g, Fat: 12g

PROTEIN ENERGY BALLS

COOKING TIME: 15 MINUTES (PLUS CHILLING TIME), SERVING: 12 BALLS

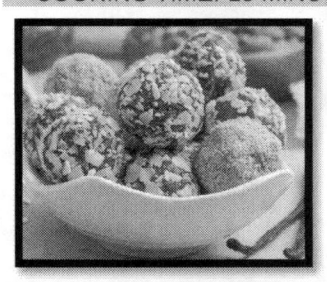

These homemade energy balls are tasty and filling. They are made with oats, almond butter, protein powder, honey, and then coated in shredded coconut.

INGREDIENTS:
- 1 cup rolled oats
- 1/2 cup almond butter
- 1/4 cup protein powder
- 1/4 cup honey
- 1/4 cup shredded coconut

STEP-BY-STEP INSTRUCTIONS:
2. Oats, almond butter, protein powder, and honey should all be thoroughly mixed in a bowl.
3. Shape into balls that are one inch in diameter.
4. Add shredded coconut and roll.
5. Place in the fridge to chill for a minimum of half an hour.

BENEFITS:

It offers long-lasting energy and is rich in protein and good fats.

NUTRITION PLAN: PER BALL

Calories: 100, Protein: 4g, Carbohydrates: 12g, Fat: 5g

SIDE DISHES

CHICKEN AND VEGETABLE SOUP

COOKING TIME: 30 MINUTES, SERVING: 4 SERVINGS

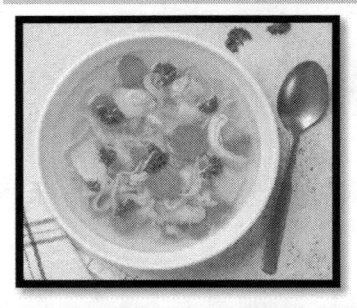

A substantial soup with mixed veggies, herbs, and diced chicken breast in a tasty broth.

INGREDIENTS:
- 1 lb chicken breast, diced
- 4 cups chicken broth
- 2 cups mixed vegetables (carrots, celery, onions)
- Two cloves garlic, minced
- One teaspoon of dried thyme
- Salt and pepper to taste

STEP-BY-STEP INSTRUCTIONS:
1. Garlic should be softened and aromatic in a big pot.
2. Cook the chopped chicken breast until it turns golden.
3. Stir in the mixed vegetables, thyme, chicken broth, salt, and pepper.
4. After 20 minutes of simmering, the vegetables should be soft.

BENEFITS:

Low in calories and high in fiber and protein.

NUTRITION PLAN: PER SERVING

Calories: 200 per serving, Protein: 25g, Carbohydrates: 10g, Fat: 5g

BROCCOLI CHEDDAR SOUP

COOKING TIME: 40 MINUTES, SERVING: 4 SERVINGS

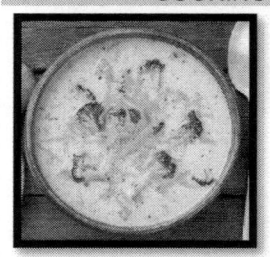

This soup is perfect for a chilly evening, with strong cheddar cheese, pureed broccoli, and a touch of nutmeg.

INGREDIENTS:
- 2 cups broccoli florets
- 2 cups chicken broth
- 1 cup shredded cheddar cheese
- 1/2 cup heavy cream
- 1/4 teaspoon nutmeg

STEP-BY-STEP INSTRUCTIONS:
1. Broccoli should be cooked in chicken stock until soft.
2. Smoothly puree the broccoli with the broth.
3. Pour cheese, cream, and nutmeg into the saucepan with the puree.
4. Simmer until the soup is thoroughly heated and the cheese has melted.

BENEFITS:

Low in carbohydrates, high in calcium and vitamin C.

NUTRITION PLAN: PER SERVING
Calories: 250, Protein: 10g, Carbohydrates: 10g, Fat: 15g

CAPRESE SALAD

COOKING TIME: 10 MINUTES, SERVING: 4 SERVINGS

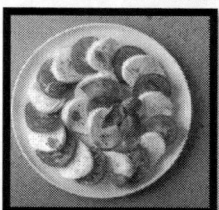

A light and delicious side dish of sliced tomatoes, fresh mozzarella, and basil leaves drizzled with balsamic sauce.

INGREDIENTS:
- Two large tomatoes, sliced
- 8 oz fresh mozzarella, sliced
- Fresh basil leaves
- Balsamic glaze for drizzling

STEP-BY-STEP INSTRUCTIONS:
1. Place slices of mozzarella and tomato on a platter.
2. Place basil leaves in between the mozzarella and tomato slices.
3. Pour balsamic glaze over.

BENEFITS:
Rich in antioxidants, calcium, and good fats.

NUTRITION PLAN: PER SERVING
Calories: 150, Protein: 10g, Carbohydrates: 5g, Fat: 10g

ROASTED BRUSSELS SPROUTS WITH BACON

COOKING TIME: 25 MINUTES, SERVING: 4 SERVINGS

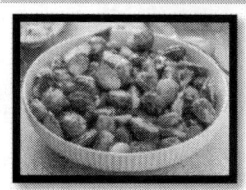

A flavorful side dish of softly roasted Brussels sprouts mixed with crunchy bacon bits and balsamic glaze.

INGREDIENTS:
- 1 lb Brussels sprouts, trimmed and halved
- Four slices bacon, cooked and crumbled
- Balsamic glaze for drizzling

STEP-BY-STEP INSTRUCTIONS:
1. Add salt, pepper, and olive oil to Brussels sprouts and toss.
2. Arrange them on a baking pan and bake at 400°F (200°C) for 20 minutes or until soft.
3. Top the roasted Brussels sprouts with crumbled cooked bacon.
4. Before serving, drizzle with balsamic glaze.

BENEFITS:
It is packed with fiber, vitamins, and antioxidants and flavored with bacon for a tasty bite.

NUTRITION PLAN: PER SERVING
Calories: 150, Protein: 8g, Carbohydrates: 10g, Fat: 8g

EGGPLANT PARMESAN

COOKING TIME: 45 MINUTES, SERVING: 4 SERVINGS

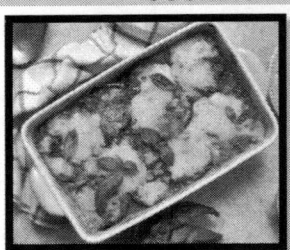

A tasty vegetarian recipe is made with sliced eggplant baked with mozzarella cheese and marinara sauce on top of a crisp almond flour crust.

INGREDIENTS:
- One large eggplant, sliced
- 1 cup almond flour
- Two eggs, beaten
- 1 cup marinara sauce
- 1 cup shredded mozzarella cheese

STEP-BY-STEP INSTRUCTIONS:
1. Coat the eggplant slices with almond flour after dipping them in beaten eggs.
2. Arrange the oiled eggplant slices onto a baking sheet and bake them for 20 minutes at 375°F (190°C).
3. Arrange baked eggplant pieces with mozzarella cheese and marinara sauce in a baking dish.
4. Bake for fifteen minutes or until the cheese is bubbling and melted.

BENEFITS:
Rich in fiber and antioxidants from eggplant, low in carbohydrates, and gluten-free.

NUTRITION PLAN: PER SERVING
Calories: 200, Protein: 10g, Carbohydrates: 15g, Fat: 10g

CUCUMBER AVOCADO SALAD

COOKING TIME: 15 MINUTES, SERVING: 4 SERVINGS

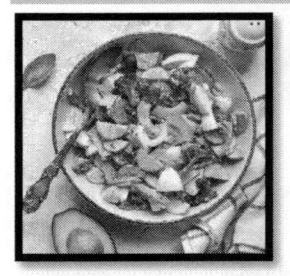

An excellent side dish consists of sliced cucumbers, creamy avocado, fresh cilantro, red onion, and zesty lime dressing.

INGREDIENTS:
- Two cucumbers, thinly sliced
- One avocado, diced
- 1/4 cup chopped fresh cilantro
- 1/4 cup diced red onion
- Juice of 1 lime
- Salt and pepper to taste

STEP-BY-STEP INSTRUCTIONS:
1. Diced avocado, red onion, cilantro, and cucumber slices should all be combined in a big bowl.
2. After drizzling the salad with lime juice, gently toss to coat.
3. To taste, add salt and pepper for seasoning.

BENEFITS:
Packed with vitamins, minerals, and good fats, the lime dressing adds a zesty kick.

NUTRITION PLAN: PER SERVING
Calories: 150, Protein: 3g, Carbohydrates: 10g, Fat: 12g

MEAL PLAN CHARTS FOR 30 DAYS

Here's a meal plan for 30 days incorporating Dr. Nowzaradan's Low Carb High Protein Recipes, with each day's total calorie intake kept under 1200 calories:

S/N	TIME	RECIPES
01	BREAKFAST	Spinach and Feta Omelette
	LUNCH	Turkey and Avocado Wrap
	DINNER	Baked Salmon with Asparagus
	SNACK	Greek Yogurt and Berry Smoothie, Roasted Chickpeas
	SIDE DISH	Cauliflower Mash
02	BREAKFAST	Crustless Quiche with Bacon and Cheddar
	LUNCH	Tuna Salad Lettuce Wraps
	DINNER	Turkey Meatballs with Zoodles
	SNACK	Cottage Cheese and Tomato Slices, Cheese and Veggie Platters
	SIDE DISH	Broccoli Cheddar Soup
03	BREAKFAST	Greek Yogurt Parfait with Berries and Almonds
	LUNCH	Zucchini Noodle Stir-Fry with Chicken
	DINNER	Spaghetti Squash with Chicken Alfredo
	SNACK	Almond Butter and Celery Sticks, Protein Energy Balls
	SIDE DISH	Caprese Salad
04	BREAKFAST	Veggie Breakfast Casserole
	LUNCH	Egg Salad Stuffed Bell Peppers
	DINNER	Beef and Broccoli Stir-Fry
	SNACK	Turkey and Cheese Roll-Ups, Roasted Brussels Sprouts with Bacon
	SIDE DISH	Eggplant Parmesan
05	BREAKFAST	Low-Carb Protein Pancakes
	LUNCH	Shrimp and Veggie Skewers
	DINNER	Stuffed Portobello Mushrooms
	SNACK	Greek Yogurt and Berry Smoothie, Roasted Chickpeas
	SIDE DISH	Grilled Asparagus with Lemon Zest
06	BREAKFAST	Smoked Salmon and Avocado Toast
	LUNCH	Cauliflower Fried Rice with Tofu
	DINNER	Grilled Lemon Herb Chicken
	SNACK	Protein-Packed Deviled Eggs, Cheese and Veggie Platters
	SIDE DISH	Chicken and Vegetable Soup
07	BREAKFAST	Cottage Cheese and Berry Bowl
	LUNCH	Greek Chicken Salad Bowl
	DINNER	Cauliflower Crust Pizza
	SNACK	Almond Butter and Celery Sticks, Cheese, and Veggie Platters
	SIDE DISH	Cucumber Avocado Salad
08	BREAKFAST	Egg and Veggie Muffin Cups
	LUNCH	Grilled Chicken Caesar Salad
	DINNER	Baked Cod with Tomato Basil Relish
	SNACK	Turkey and Cheese Roll-Ups, Roasted Chickpeas
	SIDE DISH	Broccoli Cheddar Soup
09	BREAKFAST	Spinach and Feta Omelette
	LUNCH	Turkey and Avocado Wrap
	DINNER	Beef and Broccoli Stir-Fry
	SNACK	Greek Yogurt and Berry Smoothie, Protein Energy Balls
	SIDE DISH	Roasted Brussels Sprouts with Bacon

10	BREAKFAST	Crustless Quiche with Bacon and Cheddar
	LUNCH	Tuna Salad Lettuce Wraps
	DINNER	Stuffed Portobello Mushrooms
	SNACK	Almond Butter and Celery Sticks, Cheese, and Veggie Platters
	SIDE DISH	Eggplant Parmesan
11	BREAKFAST	Greek Yogurt Parfait with Berries and Almonds
	LUNCH	Zucchini Noodle Stir-Fry with Chicken
	DINNER	Grilled Lemon Herb Chicken
	SNACK	Cottage Cheese and Tomato Slices, Roasted Chickpeas
	SIDE DISH	Grilled Asparagus with Lemon Zest
12	BREAKFAST	Veggie Breakfast Casserole
	LUNCH	Egg Salad Stuffed Bell Peppers
	DINNER	Cauliflower Crust Pizza
	SNACK	Greek Yogurt and Berry Smoothie, Protein-Packed Deviled Eggs
	SIDE DISH	Chicken and Vegetable Soup
13	BREAKFAST	Low-Carb Protein Pancakes
	LUNCH	Shrimp and Veggie Skewers
	DINNER	Baked Salmon with Asparagus
	SNACK	Almond Butter and Celery Sticks, Cheese, and Veggie Platters
	SIDE DISH	Cauliflower Mash
14	BREAKFAST	Smoked Salmon and Avocado Toast
	LUNCH	Cauliflower Fried Rice with Tofu
	DINNER	Turkey Meatballs with Zoodles
	SNACK	Greek Yogurt and Berry Smoothie, Roasted Chickpeas
	SIDE DISH	Caprese Salad
15	BREAKFAST	Cottage Cheese and Berry Bowl
	LUNCH	Greek Chicken Salad Bowl
	DINNER	Spaghetti Squash with Chicken Alfredo
	SNACK	Turkey and Cheese Roll-Ups, Roasted Chickpeas
	SIDE DISH	Roasted Brussels Sprouts with Bacon
16	BREAKFAST	Egg and Veggie Muffin Cups
	LUNCH	Grilled Chicken Caesar Salad
	DINNER	Beef and Broccoli Stir-Fry
	SNACK	Greek Yogurt and Berry Smoothie, Protein Energy Balls
	SIDE DISH	Cauliflower Mash
17	BREAKFAST	Spinach and Feta Omelette
	LUNCH	Turkey and Avocado Wrap
	DINNER	Stuffed Portobello Mushrooms
	SNACK	Almond Butter and Celery Sticks, Cheese, and Veggie Platters
	SIDE DISH	Eggplant Parmesan
18	BREAKFAST	Crustless Quiche with Bacon and Cheddar
	LUNCH	Tuna Salad Lettuce Wraps
	DINNER	Grilled Lemon Herb Chicken
	SNACK	Cottage Cheese and Tomato Slices, Roasted Chickpeas
	SIDE DISH	Grilled Asparagus with Lemon Zest
19	BREAKFAST	Greek Yogurt Parfait with Berries and Almonds
	LUNCH	Zucchini Noodle Stir-Fry with Chicken
	DINNER	Cauliflower Crust Pizza
	SNACK	Greek Yogurt and Berry Smoothie, Protein-Packed Deviled Eggs
	SIDE DISH	Chicken and Vegetable Soup
20	BREAKFAST	Veggie Breakfast Casserole
	LUNCH	Egg Salad Stuffed Bell Peppers

	DINNER	Baked Salmon with Asparagus
	SNACK	Almond Butter and Celery Sticks, Cheese, and Veggie Platters
	SIDE DISH	Caprese Salad
21	BREAKFAST	Low-Carb Protein Pancakes
	LUNCH	Shrimp and Veggie Skewers
	DINNER	Turkey Meatballs with Zoodles
	SNACK	Greek Yogurt and Berry Smoothie, Roasted Chickpeas
	SIDE DISH	Cauliflower Mash
22	BREAKFAST	Smoked Salmon and Avocado Toast
	LUNCH	Cauliflower Fried Rice with Tofu
	DINNER	Grilled Lemon Herb Chicken
	SNACK	Greek Yogurt and Berry Smoothie, Protein Energy Balls
	SIDE DISH	Grilled Asparagus with Lemon Zest
23	BREAKFAST	Cottage Cheese and Berry Bowl
	LUNCH	Greek Chicken Salad Bowl
	DINNER	Spaghetti Squash with Chicken Alfredo
	SNACK	Turkey and Cheese Roll-Ups, Roasted Chickpeas
	SIDE DISH	Roasted Brussels Sprouts with Bacon
24	BREAKFAST	Egg and Veggie Muffin Cups
	LUNCH	Grilled Chicken Caesar Salad
	DINNER	Beef and Broccoli Stir-Fry
	SNACK	Greek Yogurt and Berry Smoothie, Protein Energy Balls
	SIDE DISH	Cauliflower Mash
25	BREAKFAST	Spinach and Feta Omelette
	LUNCH	Turkey and Avocado Wrap
	DINNER	Stuffed Portobello Mushrooms
	SNACK	Almond Butter and Celery Sticks, Cheese, and Veggie Platters
	SIDE DISH	Eggplant Parmesan
26	BREAKFAST	Crustless Quiche with Bacon and Cheddar
	LUNCH	Tuna Salad Lettuce Wraps
	DINNER	Grilled Lemon Herb Chicken
	SNACK	Cottage Cheese and Tomato Slices, Roasted Chickpeas
	SIDE DISH	Grilled Asparagus with Lemon Zest
27	BREAKFAST	Greek Yogurt Parfait with Berries and Almonds
	LUNCH	Zucchini Noodle Stir-Fry with Chicken
	DINNER	Cauliflower Crust Pizza
	SNACK	Greek Yogurt and Berry Smoothie, Protein-Packed Deviled Eggs
	SIDE DISH	Chicken and Vegetable Soup
28	BREAKFAST	Veggie Breakfast Casserole
	LUNCH	Egg Salad Stuffed Bell Peppers
	DINNER	Baked Salmon with Asparagus
	SNACK	Almond Butter and Celery Sticks, Cheese, and Veggie Platters
	SIDE DISH	Caprese Salad
29	BREAKFAST	Low-Carb Protein Pancakes
	LUNCH	Shrimp and Veggie Skewers
	DINNER	Turkey Meatballs with Zoodles
	SNACK	Greek Yogurt and Berry Smoothie, Roasted Chickpeas
	SIDE DISH	Cauliflower Mash
30	BREAKFAST	Smoked Salmon and Avocado Toast
	LUNCH	Cauliflower Fried Rice with Tofu
	DINNER	Grilled Lemon Herb Chicken
	SNACK	Greek Yogurt and Berry Smoothie, Protein Energy Balls
	SIDE DISH	Grilled Asparagus with Lemon Zest

LOW-CALORIE KETO RECIPES

Welcome to the world of keto dishes low in calories! We will delve into a variety of tasty and filling meals in this book that follow the guidelines of the ketogenic diet while being low in calories. These recipes will keep you on track while allowing you to enjoy tasty meals whether you want to lose weight or live a better lifestyle.

KETOGENIC DIET OVERVIEW

The ketogenic diet is a low-carb, moderate-protein, high-fat eating regimen that compels the body to use fat for energy instead of carbs. When the body consumes a significant amount of healthy fats instead of carbohydrates, it enters a state known as ketosis, which increases its ability to burn fat for energy. This metabolic state has been linked to several health advantages, such as reduced body weight, better blood sugar regulation, and increased mental acuity.

BENEFITS OF LOW-CALORIE KETO RECIPES:
Weight Loss: These meals can help lose weight without compromising flavor or satisfaction by cutting back on carbs and emphasizing low-calorie, nutrient-dense foods.
Enhanced Energy: Research indicates that the ketogenic diet can give a consistent energy source by balancing blood sugar levels and minimizing energy swings over the day.
Enhanced Mental Clarity: Because ketones provide a steady energy source, many people who follow a ketogenic diet report having better focus, concentration, and mental clarity.
Appetite Control: These recipes' high fat and protein content will help you feel full and satisfied for longer, lowering the chance of overeating or nibbling between meals.
Blood Sugar Regulation: These recipes can help stabilize blood sugar levels by reducing the amount of carbohydrates consumed, which may be advantageous for those with diabetes or insulin resistance.

Let's start with these delectable low-calorie keto dishes, which will satisfy your palate and help you reach your wellness and health objectives!

INTRODUCTION TO THE KETOGENIC DIET

Here, you can learn about the ketogenic diet, a nutritional strategy that has become very popular due to its possible health advantages and ability to help people lose weight. This introduction will cover the basics of the ketogenic diet, its guiding ideas, and its potential effects on your health and well-being.

WHAT IS THE KETOGENIC DIET?
A high-fat, moderate-protein, low-carb diet, often known as the ketogenic diet, is intended to cause the body to enter a state of ketosis through altered metabolism. As an alternative fuel source to glucose received from carbohydrates, the body creates ketones during ketosis from fat storage. The ketogenic diet seeks to cause the body to burn fat more effectively for energy by sharply lowering carbohydrate intake and raising fat consumption. This can result in weight loss and other health advantages.

KEY PRINCIPLES OF THE KETOGENIC DIET:

Minimal Carbohydrate Intake: Depending on personal variables, including age, weight, and degree of activity, the ketogenic diet usually limits daily carbohydrate consumption to 20–50 grams. Ketosis is a metabolic state in which the body burns fat for energy, requiring this limitation to be induced and maintained.

Moderate Protein Consumption: Although protein is a necessary macronutrient for repairing muscles and other body processes, too much protein might disrupt ketosis by converting to glucose through a process known as gluconeogenesis. The ketogenic diet strongly emphasizes moderate protein consumption to avoid producing too much glucose.

High Intake of Fat: Between 70 and 80 percent of daily calories on a ketogenic diet come from fat. For satiety and long-lasting energy, it's recommended to consume healthy, fat-containing foods such as fatty fish, avocados, nuts, seeds, and olive oil.

Ketosis: When the body burns fat for energy efficiently, it enters a metabolic condition known as ketosis, defined by elevated blood ketone levels. One of the main objectives of the ketogenic diet is to achieve and sustain ketosis, which can be seen with breath ketone analyzers, blood ketone meters, and urine strips.

HEALTH BENEFITS OF THE KETOGENIC DIET

Beyond helping people lose weight, the ketogenic diet has been linked to several health advantages, such as:

Weight Loss: The ketogenic diet can significantly reduce appetite and promote fat burning, which is especially beneficial for people who are obese or have excess body fat.

Better Blood Sugar Control: The ketogenic diet may benefit people with type 2 diabetes or prediabetes as a therapeutic strategy, helping them control their blood sugar levels and increase their insulin sensitivity.

Enhanced Mental Clarity: Due to the ketogenic diet's consistent delivery of ketones to the brain, many people report improved attention, mental clarity, and cognitive function.

Enhanced Energy: The ketogenic diet offers a steady supply of energy by using fat reserves as fuel, minimizing the swings in energy that are frequently associated with diets high in carbohydrates.

Decreased Inflammation: Some research suggests that the ketogenic diet may have anti-inflammatory properties, which could be advantageous for people who suffer from autoimmune illnesses or other conditions associated with chronic inflammation
, like arthritis.

Like with any dietary plan, it is imperative to speak with a healthcare provider before beginning the ketogenic diet, particularly if you are taking medication or have underlying medical conditions. Furthermore, each person will react differently to the ketogenic diet. Therefore, paying attention to your body and modifying your food intake is essential.

BENEFITS OF THE KETO DIET

Beyond weight reduction, the ketogenic diet, sometimes known as the "keto diet," has drawn interest due to its possible health advantages. Let's examine a few of the main benefits of embracing a ketogenic lifestyle:

WEIGHT LOSS:
One of the ketogenic diet's best-known advantages is its ability to help people lose weight. The diet assists the body in entering a state of ketosis, when it burns stored fat for energy, by limiting the amount of carbohydrates consumed and encouraging the ingestion of healthy fats and enough protein. This can result in notable weight losses, especially for those who are obese or have extra body fat.

BETTER BLOOD SUGAR CONTROL:
Research has indicated that the ketogenic diet may help those with type 2 diabetes or prediabetes by raising insulin sensitivity and blood sugar levels. By limiting the amount of carbohydrates consumed and stabilizing blood sugar levels, the diet may help control insulin production and lower the risk of blood sugar spikes and crashes.

IMPROVED FOCUS AND MENTAL CLARITY:
Many people who follow a ketogenic diet report improved focus, mental clarity, and cognitive performance. This is believed to be caused by the brain's constant supply of ketones, a more reliable and effective energy source than glucose. It has been demonstrated that ketones promote brain health and may have neuroprotective properties.

SUSTAINED ENERGY LEVELS:
The ketogenic diet offers a steady supply of energy all day long since it uses fat as fuel rather than carbohydrates. People in ketosis benefit from a more constant and continuous energy source, which helps them feel more focused, alert, and energized than those who follow diets high in carbohydrates, which frequently cause energy fluctuations.

HUNGER CONTROL AND DECREASED DESIRES:
People who follow a ketogenic diet may naturally cut back on calories and lessen their desires for items high in sugar and carbohydrates. This is because the diet is well-known for its ability to suppress hunger. Keto meals' high fat and moderate protein content helps people feel full and avoid hunger, which makes it simpler to follow a diet low in calories.

CARDIOVASCULAR HEALTH:
Despite having a high content of saturated fats, studies have indicated that the ketogenic diet can enhance blood pressure, HDL (the "good") cholesterol, triglyceride levels, and other cardiovascular health markers. Further study is necessary to corroborate the findings of several studies that suggest the keto diet may help lower the risk of heart disease and stroke.

POTENTIAL ANTI-INFLAMMATORY EFFECTS:
Heart disease, diabetes, and autoimmune disorders are just a few of the illnesses that have been connected to the development of chronic inflammation. According to specific research, the ketogenic diet has anti-inflammatory properties that lower bodily inflammation and the risk of inflammatory illnesses.

METABOLIC FLEXIBILITY:
A ketogenic diet improves metabolic flexibility, enabling the body to switch between burning fat and carbohydrates for energy efficiently. This metabolic adaptation may enhance overall metabolic health and resilience by decreasing the risk of metabolic illnesses, including insulin resistance and metabolic syndrome.

It's crucial to remember that not everyone will benefit from or respond to the ketogenic diet similarly. Furthermore, research is still being done on the long-term health effects of sustained ketosis, so it's imperative to speak with a healthcare provider before beginning any new diet or lifestyle plan, particularly if you have any underlying medical illnesses or concerns.

KETO BREAKFAST RECIPES

SPINACH AND MUSHROOM CRUSTLESS QUICHE

COOKING TIME: 45 MINUTES, SERVING: 6 SERVINGS

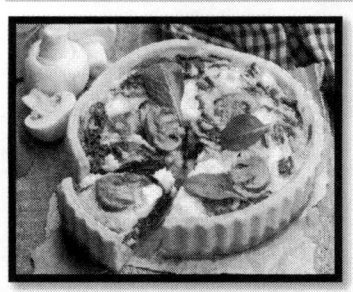

A flavorful quiche made with eggs, spinach, mushrooms, and a touch of cheese, baked to perfection without the crust.

INGREDIENTS:
- Six large eggs
- 1 cup chopped spinach
- 1 cup sliced mushrooms
- 1/2 cup shredded cheese (cheddar or mozzarella)
- Salt and pepper to taste

STEP-BY-STEP INSTRUCTIONS:
1. Turn the oven on to 375°F, or 190°C. Apply grease to a pie dish.
2. Whisk the eggs in a bowl. Add pepper and salt for seasoning.
3. Add the sliced mushrooms, shredded cheese, and chopped spinach and stir.
4. Fill the prepared pie dish with the mixture.
5. The quiche should bake for 25 to 30 minutes or until the top is golden brown and set.
6. Let it cool down a little before cutting and serving.

BENEFITS:
It is packed with vitamins and minerals from spinach and mushrooms, low in carbohydrates, high in protein and fiber.

NUTRITION PLAN: PER SERVING
Calories: 150, Protein: 10g, Carbohydrates: 3g, Fat: 10g

KETO AVOCADO EGG CUPS

COOKING TIME: 20 MINUTES, SERVING: 4 SERVINGS

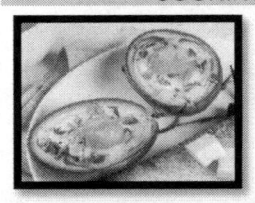

A tasty breakfast meal is made by filling halved avocados with broken eggs and baking until the eggs are set.

INGREDIENTS:
- Two ripe avocados
- Four eggs
- Salt and pepper to taste

STEP-BY-STEP INSTRUCTIONS:
1. Turn the oven on to 375°F, or 190°C. Halve the avocados and scoop out the pits.
2. To create room for the egg, scoop away a tiny amount of additional flesh from each avocado half.
3. In each half of an avocado, crack one egg. Add pepper and salt for seasoning.
4. Once the eggs are set, place the avocado halves on a baking sheet and bake for 12 to 15 minutes.
5. If desired, top the hot dish with more seasoning.

BENEFITS:
It is low in carbohydrates, fiber, protein, and healthy fats, making it a breakfast option suitable for ketogenic diets.

NUTRITION PLAN: PER SERVING
Calories: 200 per serving. Protein: 8g. Carbohydrates: 5g. Fat: 15g

ZUCCHINI FRITTERS WITH SOUR CREAM

COOKING TIME: 30 MINUTES, SERVING: 4 SERVINGS

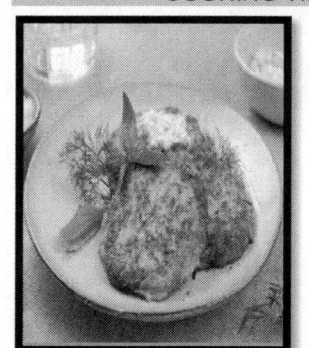

They were then pan-fried till golden brown and served with a dollop of sour cream.

INGREDIENTS:
- Two medium zucchinis, grated
- Two eggs
- 1/4 cup almond flour
- 1/4 cup grated Parmesan cheese
- Two cloves garlic, minced
- One tablespoon of chopped fresh parsley
- Salt and pepper to taste
- Olive oil for frying
- Sour cream for serving

STEP-BY-STEP INSTRUCTIONS:
1. After grating the zucchini, place it in a fresh kitchen towel and remove any extra moisture.
2. Squeezed zucchini, eggs, almond flour, Parmesan cheese, minced garlic, chopped parsley, salt, and pepper should all be combined in a big basin. Blend until thoroughly blended.
3. In a skillet over medium heat, warm the olive oil.
4. Form the zucchini mixture into patties using a 1/4 cup scoop. After placing them in the skillet, gently flatten the patties using a spatula.
5. Fry for 3–4 minutes on each side or until crispy and golden brown.

6. Top each hot serving of zucchini fritters with a dollop of sour cream.

BENEFITS:
Made with almond flour and zucchini, these cakes are low in carbohydrates, high in fiber and protein, and nutrient-dense.

NUTRITION PLAN: PER SERVING
Calories: 120, Protein: 6g, Carbohydrates: 6g, Fat: 8g

EGG AND BACON MUFFIN CUPS

COOKING TIME: 25 MINUTES, SERVING: 6 SERVINGS

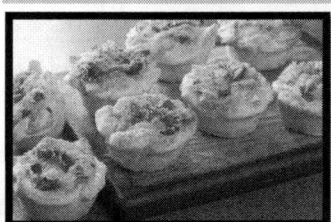

A quick and portable breakfast option is made with whisked eggs, fried bacon bits, and minced chives baked in muffin pans.

INGREDIENTS:
- Six large eggs
- Four slices bacon, cooked and crumbled
- Two tablespoons chopped chives
- Salt and pepper to taste

STEP-BY-STEP INSTRUCTIONS:
1. Set the oven's temperature to 175°C/350°F. Use paper liners or grease a muffin pan.
2. Beat the eggs until they are well-beaten in a bowl. Add pepper and salt for seasoning.
3. Add the chopped chives and fried bacon bits and stir.
4. The egg mixture should fill each cup of the prepared muffin tray about 3/4 of the way to the top.
5. Bake the muffin cups for 15 to 18 minutes or until they are firm and have a hint of color on top.
6. Before removing it from the muffin tray, let it cool somewhat. Heat or serve at room temperature.

BENEFITS:
These protein-rich, low-carb muffin cups are ideal for meal prep or quick meals.

NUTRITION PLAN: PER SERVING
Calories: 150, Protein: 10g, Carbohydrates: 1g, Fat: 11g

KETO GREEN SMOOTHIE

COOKING TIME: 5 MINUTES, SERVING: 2 SERVINGS

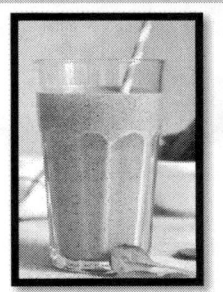

Smooth and creamy spinach, avocado, cucumber, coconut milk, and a scoop of protein powder are mixed to create this energizing smoothie.

INGREDIENTS:
- 2 cups spinach leaves
- 1/2 ripe avocado
- 1/2 cucumber, peeled and chopped
- 1 cup unsweetened coconut milk
- One scoop of vanilla protein powder
- Ice cubes (optional)

STEP-BY-STEP INSTRUCTIONS:
1. Put the spinach, cucumber, avocado, coconut milk, and protein powder in a blender.
2. If you want your smoothie colder, add a few ice cubes.
3. Process quickly until smooth and creamy; adjust consistency with additional coconut milk if needed.
4. After transferring the smoothie into glasses, serve it right away.

BENEFITS:
Packed with fiber, healthy fats, and protein, this smoothie is an excellent choice for a nutrient-dense breakfast or post-workout snack.

NUTRITION PLAN: PER SERVING
Calories: 200 per serving, Protein: 15g, Carbohydrates: 8g, Fat: 12g

ALMOND FLOUR PANCAKES WITH BERRIES
COOKING TIME: 15 MINUTES, SERVING: 4 SERVINGS

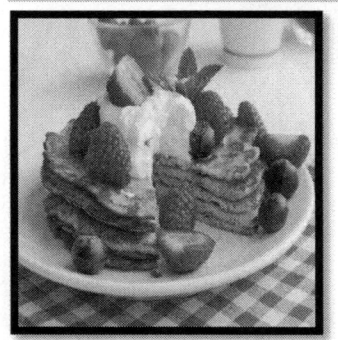

A guilt-free breakfast treat of fluffy pancakes cooked.

INGREDIENTS:
- 1 cup almond flour
- Two large eggs
- 1/4 cup unsweetened almond milk
- One tablespoon of granulated sweetener
- One teaspoon of baking powder
- 1/2 teaspoon vanilla extract
- Pinch of salt
- Cooking spray or butter for greasing the pan
- Mixed berries and sugar-free syrup for serving

STEP-BY-STEP INSTRUCTIONS:
1. If using sweetener, gently mix almond flour, eggs, almond milk, baking powder, vanilla extract, and salt in a mixing dish.
2. Grease a non-stick skillet or griddle with cooking spray or butter and heat it over medium heat.
3. Transfer approximately 1/4 cup of the batter onto the skillet for each pancake.
4. Cook the pancakes until bubbles appear on their surface, then turn them over and continue cooking until the second side is golden brown.
5. Grease the skillet as necessary and repeat with the remaining batter.
6. Top the pancakes with a mixture of berries and a thin layer of sugar-free syrup, and serve.

BENEFITS:
These pancakes are a tasty and wholesome choice for a ketogenic breakfast because they are low in carbohydrates, rich in protein, and high in healthy fats. They are also gluten-free.

NUTRITION PLAN: PER SERVING
Calories: 180 per serving, Protein: 8g, Carbohydrates: 6g, Fat: 14g

KETO LUNCH RECIPES

KETO CHICKEN SALAD LETTUCE WRAPS

COOKING TIME: 15 MINUTES, SERVING: 4 SERVINGS

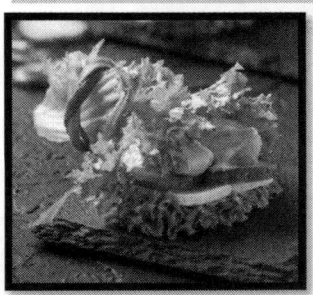

Serve shredded chicken with mayonnaise, sliced almonds, and diced celery on crisp lettuce leaves for a light and energizing meal.

INGREDIENTS:
- 2 cups cooked shredded chicken breast
- 1/4 cup mayonnaise
- 1/4 cup diced celery
- 1/4 cup chopped almonds
- Salt and pepper to taste
- Large lettuce leaves for serving

STEP-BY-STEP INSTRUCTIONS:
1. Add the chopped almonds, diced celery, mayonnaise, and shredded chicken to a mixing bowl.
2. Toss to mix in the salt and pepper, if desired thoroughly.
3. Place a spoonful of the chicken salad mixture in the middle of each lettuce
4. leaf.
5. Roll up the leaves and fasten with toothpicks to make lettuce wraps.
6. Serve immediately or put in the fridge until you're ready to eat.

BENEFITS:
These lettuce wraps are an excellent choice for a keto-friendly lunch because they are high in protein, low in carbohydrates, and flavorful.

NUTRITION PLAN: PER SERVING
Calories: 250, Protein: 20g, Carbohydrates: 3g, Fat: 18g

KETO TURKEY CLUB LETTUCE WRAPS

COOKING TIME: 15 MINUTES, SERVING: 4 SERVINGS

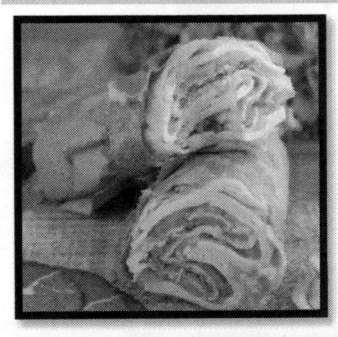

A low-carb take on the traditional club sandwich: sliced turkey breast wrapped in big lettuce leaves and piled with crispy bacon, avocado slices, lettuce, and tomato.

INGREDIENTS:
- 1 lb sliced turkey breast
- Eight slices of cooked bacon
- One avocado, sliced
- Four large lettuce leaves
- One tomato, sliced
- Mayonnaise (optional)

STEP-BY-STEP INSTRUCTIONS:
1. Arrange the lettuce leaves on a spotlessly tidy tabletop.
2. Sliced turkey breast, cooked bacon, avocado, tomato, and, if you like, a dollop of mayonnaise should be added to the top of each lettuce leaf.
3. To make lettuce wraps, roll up the leaves.
4. If necessary, fasten with toothpicks and serve right away.

BENEFITS:
Ideal for a keto lunch, these lettuce wraps are a tasty way to get all the flavors of a traditional club sandwich without the added carbohydrates.

NUTRITION PLAN: PER SERVING
Calories: 280 per serving, Protein: 25g, Carbohydrates: 4g, Fat: 18g

KETO TACO SALAD

COOKING TIME: 20 MINUTES, SERVING: 4 SERVINGS

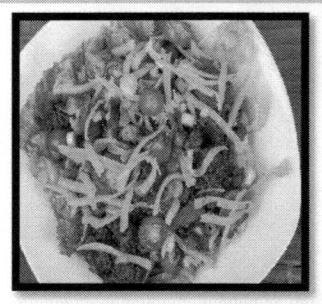

A filling Tex-Mex-inspired lunch would consist of seasoned ground beef cooked with taco seasoning

INGREDIENTS:
- 1 lb ground beef
- One packet of taco seasoning (low-carb if possible)
- 4 cups mixed greens
- 1 cup shredded cheddar cheese
- One avocado, diced
- 1 cup salsa

STEP-BY-STEP INSTRUCTIONS:
1. The ground beef should be cooked in a skillet over medium heat. Eliminate extra fat.
2. As directed on the packet, add the taco seasoning to the beef.
3. Arrange the mixed greens in a big bowl.
4. Add salsa, diced avocado, shredded cheese, and seasoned ground meat.
5. Serve right away.

BENEFITS:
This taco salad is a wholesome and keto-friendly supper since it has a perfect ratio of vegetables, healthy fats, and protein.

NUTRITION PLAN: PER SERVING
Calories: 400, Protein: 30g, Carbohydrates: 7g, Fat: 28g

KETO EGG ROLL IN A BOWL

COOKING TIME: 25 MINUTES, SERVING: 4 SERVINGS

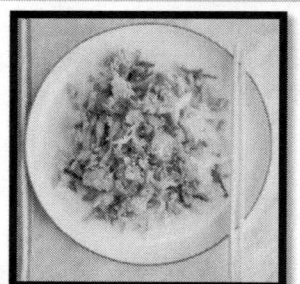

A deconstructed egg roll experience without the wrapper is achieved

INGREDIENTS:
- 1 lb ground pork
- 4 cups shredded cabbage
- 1 cup shredded carrots
- One onion, diced
- Two cloves garlic, minced
- 1 tbsp ginger, minced
- 1/4 cup soy sauce (or tamari for gluten-free)

STEP-BY-STEP INSTRUCTIONS:
1. Cook the ground pork in a big skillet over medium heat until it's browned. Eliminate extra fat.

2. To the skillet, add the ginger, garlic, and onion. Cook the onion until it becomes transparent.
3. Add the carrots and the shredded cabbage. Sauté the veggies until they are soft.
4. After adding the soy sauce, simmer for two to three minutes.
5. Warm up the food.

BENEFITS:
This dish is ideal for a ketogenic diet because it's a quick and straightforward way to experience the flavors of an egg roll without the added carbohydrates.

NUTRITION PLAN: PER SERVING
Calories: 320, Protein: 22g, Carbohydrates: 10g, Fat: 22g

KETO CAULIFLOWER FRIED RICE
COOKING TIME: 20 MINUTES, SERVING: 4 SERVINGS

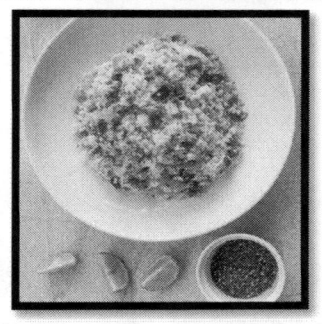

A tasty and low-carb substitute for typical fried rice is riced cauliflower stir-fried with diced vegetables, scrambled eggs, and tamari sauce.

INGREDIENTS:
- One head cauliflower, riced
- 1 cup mixed diced vegetables (carrots, peas, bell peppers)
- Two eggs, beaten
- 2 tbsp tamari sauce
- Two cloves garlic, minced
- 1 tbsp sesame oil

STEP-BY-STEP INSTRUCTIONS:
1. In a large skillet over medium heat, warm the sesame oil.
2. Garlic is added and cooked until aromatic.
3. Cook for approximately five minutes or until the riced cauliflower is soft.
4. Add the beaten eggs to the skillet after pushing the cauliflower to the side. Cook the eggs through by scrambling them.
5. Add the tamari sauce and mixed vegetables and stir. Simmer for a further three to four minutes.
6. Warm up the food.

BENEFITS:
This recipe is a fantastic high-fiber, low-carb substitute for regular fried rice appropriate for a ketogenic diet.

NUTRITION PLAN: PER SERVING
Calories: 150, Protein: 7g, Carbohydrates: 8g, Fat: 10g

KETO AVOCADO TUNA SALAD

COOKING TIME: 10 MINUTES, SERVING: 2 SERVINGS

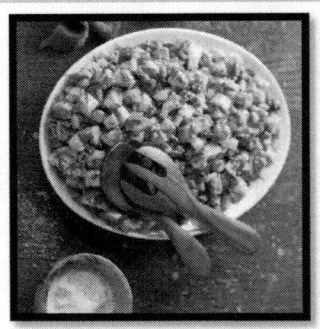

A filling and light lunch choice would be chunky tuna mixed

INGREDIENTS:
- One can (5 oz) tuna, drained
- One avocado, mashed
- 1/4 cup diced cucumber
- 2 tbsp diced red onion
- 1 tbsp lemon juice
- 1 tsp fresh dill, chopped
- Salt and pepper to taste
- Lettuce leaves for serving

STEP-BY-STEP INSTRUCTIONS:
1. Tuna, sliced cucumber, red onion, and mashed avocado should all be combined in a mixing dish.
2. Add the salt, pepper, lemon juice, and fresh dill. Blend thoroughly.
3. Place a bed of lettuce leaves on which to serve the tuna salad.

BENEFITS:
This salad is a terrific choice for a keto-friendly dinner because it's high in protein and healthy fats.

NUTRITION PLAN: PER SERVING
Calories: 250, Protein: 18g, Carbohydrates: 6g, Fat: 18g

KETO TURKEY AND CHEESE ROLL-UPS

COOKING TIME: 10 MINUTES, SERVING: 2 SERVINGS

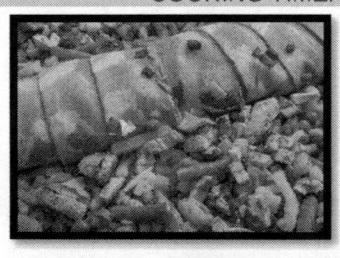

An effortless keto-friendly meal may be made by rolling sliced turkey breast with cream cheese and baby spinach leaves and fastening it with toothpicks.

INGREDIENTS:
- Eight slices of turkey breast
- 4 tbsp cream cheese
- 1 cup baby spinach leaves

STEP-BY-STEP INSTRUCTIONS:
1. Arrange the pieces of turkey on a sanitized surface.
2. On each slice of turkey, spread cream cheese.
3. Add baby spinach leaves on top.
4. Each slice of turkey is rolled up and fastened with toothpicks.
5. Serve right away.

BENEFITS:
These roll-ups are an easy and quick way to eat a low-carb, high-protein snack or supper.

NUTRITION PLAN: PER SERVING
Calories: 200, Protein: 18g, Carbohydrates: 3g, Fat: 12g

KETO GREEK SALAD WITH GRILLED CHICKEN

COOKING TIME: 30 MINUTES, SERVING: 4 SERVINGS

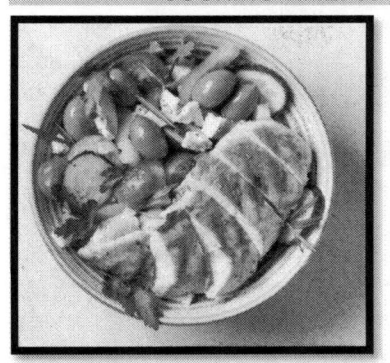

Grilled chicken breast is placed on top of crisp romaine lettuce mixed

INGREDIENTS:

- Two chicken breasts
- 4 cups romaine lettuce, chopped
- One cucumber, sliced
- 1 cup cherry tomatoes, halved
- 1/2 cup Kalamata olives
- 1/2 cup crumbled feta cheese
- 2 tbsp olive oil
- 1 tbsp lemon juice
- Salt and pepper to taste

STEP-BY-STEP INSTRUCTIONS:

1. Add salt and pepper to the chicken breasts for seasoning. Place on the grill and cook until done.
2. Toss the romaine lettuce, cucumber, cherry tomatoes, olives, and feta cheese in a big bowl.
3. The grilled chicken should be sliced and added to the salad.
4. Pour in some lemon juice and olive oil. To mix, toss.
5. Serve right away.

BENEFITS:

Packed with healthy fats and protein, this salad is a filling and nutritious keto-friendly dish.

NUTRITION PLAN: PER SERVING

Calories: 350, Protein: 30g, Carbohydrates: 8g, Fat: 22g

KETO DINNER RECIPES

KETO BAKED SALMON WITH LEMON BUTTER SAUCE

COOKING TIME: 25 MINUTES, SERVING: 4 SERVINGS

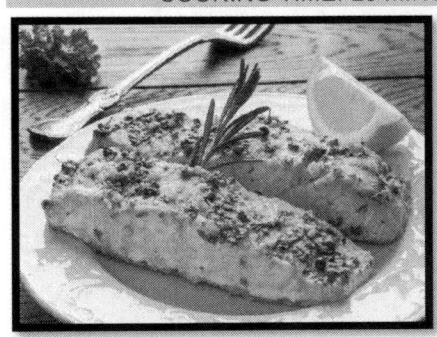

Perfectly cooked and served with a thick, tart lemon butter sauce, this keto-friendly salmon meal is seasoned with fresh herbs and lemon zest.

INGREDIENTS:

- Four salmon fillets
- 2 tbsp olive oil
- One lemon (zested and juiced)
- 2 tsp fresh dill (chopped)
- Salt and pepper to taste
- 4 tbsp butter
- Two cloves garlic (minced)

STEP-BY-STEP INSTRUCTIONS:

1. Turn the oven on to 375°F, or 190°C.
2. Arrange the salmon fillets on a parchment paper-lined baking pan.
3. Pour olive oil onto the fish and season with salt, pepper, dill, and lemon zest.
4. Bake the salmon for 15 to 20 minutes or until it is tender.
5. Melt butter in a small pot over a medium heat. When aromatic, add the garlic and simmer.
6. Cook for an additional minute after adding the lemon juice.
7. To serve, drizzle the cooked salmon with the lemon butter sauce.

BENEFITS:
They are packed with high-quality protein and omega-3 fatty acids, which support heart health and muscle maintenance.

NUTRITION PLAN: PER SERVING
Calories: 350, Protein: 25g, Fat: 27g, Carbohydrates: 2g

KETO CAULIFLOWER CRUST PIZZA

COOKING TIME: 45 MINUTES, SERVING: 4 SERVINGS

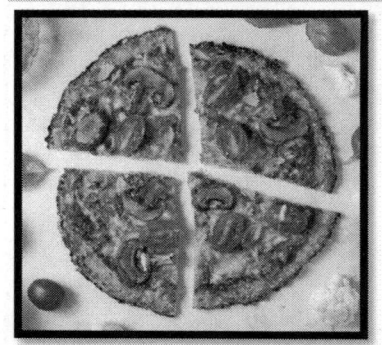

A cauliflower crust low-carb pizza that will satisfy your appetites for pizza without adding too many extra carbohydrates.

INGREDIENTS:
- One medium cauliflower (riced)
- 1 cup shredded mozzarella cheese
- 1/4 cup grated Parmesan cheese
- One large egg
- 1 tsp Italian seasoning
- 1/2 cup marinara sauce
- Additional toppings (pepperoni, vegetables, etc.)

STEP-BY-STEP INSTRUCTIONS:
1. Aim for 425°F (220°C) in the oven.
2. After the cauliflower rice is soft from steam, drain it and use a fresh towel to remove any remaining moisture.
3. Mix the cauliflower, egg, Parmesan, mozzarella, and Italian seasoning in a bowl.
4. Press the mixture onto a baking sheet lined with parchment paper to form a crust.
5. Roast for 15 to 20 minutes or until browned on top.
6. After covering the crust with marinara sauce, top with your preferred ingredients.
7. Bake for ten more minutes until the cheese is bubbling and melted.

BENEFITS:
It's a terrific substitute for regular pizza crust because it's substantial in fiber and low in carbohydrates.

NUTRITION PLAN: PER SERVING
Calories: 200, Protein: 12g, Fat: 12g, Carbohydrates: 8g

KETO GARLIC BUTTER SHRIMP SCAMPI

COOKING TIME: 20 MINUTES, SERVING: 4 SERVINGS

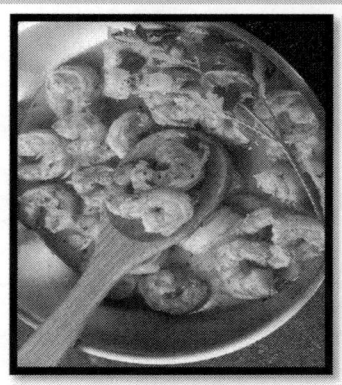

Serve luscious shrimp cooked in a garlic butter sauce over spaghetti squash or zucchini noodles for a quick and delectable keto dinner.

INGREDIENTS:
- 1 lb shrimp (peeled and deveined)
- 4 tbsp butter
- Four cloves garlic (minced)
- 1/4 cup chicken broth
- One lemon (juiced)
- 1/4 tsp red pepper flakes
- Salt and pepper to taste
- Two zucchinis (spiralized into noodles) or one spaghetti squash

STEP-BY-STEP INSTRUCTIONS:
1. Melt butter in a big skillet over a medium heat. When aromatic, add the garlic and simmer.
2. Add the shrimp and season with the red pepper flakes, salt, and pepper. Cook until all of the shrimp is cooked through and pink.
3. Add the lemon juice and chicken broth, then boil for a few minutes.
4. Add the spaghetti squash or zucchini noodles and heat thoroughly.
5. Serve right away.

BENEFITS:
Rich in fiber from the veggie noodles and high in protein and healthful fats.

NUTRITION PLAN: PER SERVING
Calories: 300, Protein: 25g, Fat: 20g Carbohydrates: 6g

KETO CHICKEN ALFREDO ZOODLES

COOKING TIME: 30 MINUTES, SERVING: 4 SERVINGS

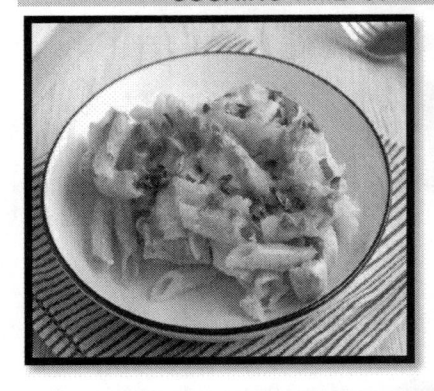

A thick Alfredo sauce combines zucchini noodles and grilled chicken to create a creamy, luscious keto pasta dish.

INGREDIENTS:
- Two large zucchinis (spiralized into noodles)
- Two chicken breasts (grilled and sliced)
- 1 cup heavy cream
- 1/2 cup Parmesan cheese (grated)
- Two cloves garlic (minced)
- Salt and pepper to taste
- 1 tbsp olive oil

STEP-BY-STEP INSTRUCTIONS:
1. Warm the olive oil in a skillet over medium heat. When aromatic, add the garlic and simmer.

2. After adding the heavy cream, boil the mixture.
3. Once the sauce thickens, stir in the Parmesan cheese. Add pepper and salt for seasoning.
4. Toss to cover in sauce, then add the grilled chicken and zucchini noodles.
5. Simmer for three to five minutes until noodles are soft but crunchy.
6. Serve right away.

BENEFITS:
Rich in protein, good fats, and low in carbohydrates, this dish makes a filling supper without the high-carb pasta.

NUTRITION PLAN: PER SERVING
Calories: 400, Protein: 30g, Fat: 30g, Carbohydrates: 8g

KETO STUFFED BELL PEPPERS
COOKING TIME: 45 MINUTES, SERVING: 4 SERVINGS

Stuffed bell peppers with a tasty blend of ground meat, spices, and cauliflower rice with melted cheese.

INGREDIENTS:
- Four bell peppers (tops cut off/seeds removed)
- 1 lb ground beef
- 1 cup cauliflower rice
- One can of diced tomatoes (drained)
- 1 cup shredded cheese
- 1 tsp chili powder
- 1 tsp cumin
- Salt and pepper to taste

STEP-BY-STEP INSTRUCTIONS:
1. Turn the oven on to 375°F, or 190°C.
2. Cook ground beef till browned in a pan. Eliminate extra
3. pepper, toes, chili powder, cumin, salt, pepper, and cauliflower rice. Cook until well heated.
4. Place the meat mixture inside bell peppers and bake them.
5. Add some shredded cheese on top.
6. Bake for 25 to 30 minutes until the cheese is melted and the peppers are soft.

BENEFITS:
This dish is packed with vitamins and minerals from the bell peppers and is an excellent source of healthy fats and protein.

NUTRITION PLAN: PER SERVING
Calories: 350, Protein: 25g, Fat: 20g, Carbohydrates: 10g

KETO BEEF AND BROCCOLI STIR-FRY

COOKING TIME: 20 MINUTES, SERVING: 4 SERVINGS

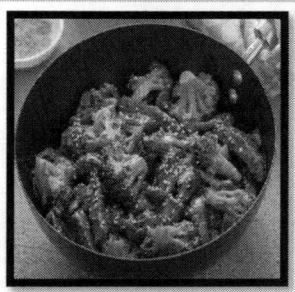

A tasty low-carb sauce pairs well with delicate meat and broccoli florets in this easy and fulfilling stir-fry.

INGREDIENTS:
- 1 lb beef sirloin (thinly sliced)
- 4 cups broccoli florets
- 3 tbsp soy sauce
- 2 tbsp olive oil
- Two cloves garlic (minced)
- 1 tsp ginger (grated)
- 1 tbsp low-carb sweetener

STEP-BY-STEP INSTRUCTIONS:
1. Heat one tablespoon of olive oil in a large skillet over medium-high heat. Add the beef and cook until it turns brown. Remove it and set it aside.
2. Add the ginger, garlic, and remaining olive oil to the skillet. Cook until aromatic.
3. Stir-fry the broccoli until it becomes crisp-tender.
4. Put the steak back in the skillet, sugar, and soy sauce. Mix thoroughly and warm through.
5. Serve right away.

BENEFITS:
Packed with fiber and protein, this dish keeps muscles firm and the digestive system healthy.

NUTRITION PLAN: PER SERVING
Calories: 300, Protein: 30g, Fat: 15g, Carbohydrates: 10g

KETO SPAGHETTI SQUASH WITH MEATBALLS

COOKING TIME: 1 HOUR, SERVING: 4 SERVINGS

A hearty, low-carb take on spaghetti and meatballs.

INGREDIENTS:
- One large spaghetti squash
- 1 lb ground beef
- 1/4 cup almond flour
- One egg
- Two cloves garlic (minced)
- 1 tsp Italian seasoning
- Salt and pepper to taste
- 2 cups marinara sauce
- 1/4 cup grated Parmesan cheese (optional)

STEP-BY-STEP INSTRUCTIONS:
1. Turn the oven on to 400°F or 200°C. After cutting the spaghetti squash in half lengthwise, remove the seeds.
2. Spread olive oil over the squash, sprinkle salt and pepper on it, and arrange it cut-side down on a baking pan—Roast until soft, about 40 minutes.

3. While the squash is roasting, combine the ground beef, almond flour, egg, garlic, Italian seasoning, salt, and pepper in a bowl and shape into meatballs.
4. Meatballs should be cooked in a large skillet over medium heat until browned all over. Simmer the meatballs in the marinara sauce until thoroughly cooked.
5. Scrape the spaghetti squash threads using a fork and divide them among plates. Add meatballs and marinara sauce on top. If preferred, sprinkle with Parmesan cheese.

BENEFITS:
This dish offers a satisfying meal that promotes muscle growth and satiety because it is high in protein and low in carbs.

NUTRITION PLAN: PER SERVING
Calories: 400, Protein: 30g, Fat: 25g, Carbohydrates: 15g

KETO SNACK RECIPES

KETO CHEESE CRISPS

COOKING TIME: 10 MINUTES, SERVING: 4 SERVINGS

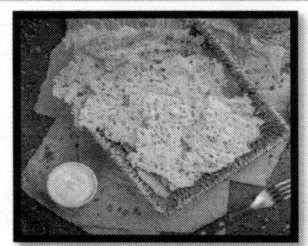

Shredded cheese is cooked until crispy and brown before cooling and cutting into bite-sized pieces for a crunchy and pleasant snack.

INGREDIENTS:
- 1 cup shredded cheese (cheddar, mozzarella, or your choice)

STEP-BY-STEP INSTRUCTIONS:
1. Preheat the oven to 375° Fahrenheit (190° Celsius).
2. Line a baking sheet with parchment paper.
3. Place small mounds of shredded cheese on the parchment paper, leaving space between them.
4. Bake for 5–7 minutes until the edges are golden and crispy.
5. Remove from the oven and allow it to cool fully.
6. Once chilled, chop or break the cheese crisps into bite-sized pieces.

BENEFITS:
Cheese crisps are high in protein and calcium, providing a delightful crunch without the carbohydrates.

NUTRITION PLAN: PER SERVING
Calories: 100, Protein: 7g, Fat: 8g, Carbohydrates: 1g

KETO GUACAMOLE WITH VEGGIE STICKS

COOKING TIME: 15 MINUTES, SERVING: 4 SERVINGS

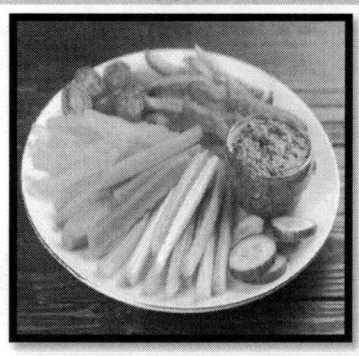

Fresh guacamole made with mashed avocado, lime juice, cilantro, and chopped tomatoes, served with sliced cucumbers, bell peppers, and celery sticks to dip.

INGREDIENTS:
- Two ripe avocados
- One lime (juiced)
- 2 tbsp chopped cilantro
- 1/4 cup diced tomatoes
- Salt and pepper to taste
- Assorted vegetable sticks (cucumber, bell peppers, celery)

STEP-BY-STEP INSTRUCTIONS:
1. Mash the avocados in a bowl with a fork until smooth.
2. Mix in the lime juice, cilantro, diced tomatoes, salt, and pepper.
3. Season to taste.
4. Serve with various veggie sticks for dipping.

BENEFITS:
Avocados and vegetables give beneficial fats, fiber, vitamins, and minerals, resulting in a nutritious and enjoyable snack.

NUTRITION PLAN: PER SERVING
Calories: 150, Protein: 2g, Fat: 12g, Carbohydrates: 9g

KETO FAT BOMBS

COOKING TIME: 15 MINUTES, SERVING: 12 SERVINGS

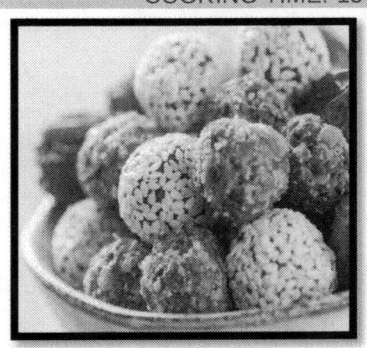

Homemade fat bombs made with coconut oil, almond butter, cocoa powder, and a low-calorie sweetener are shaped into bite-sized balls for a rapid energy boost.

INGREDIENTS:
- 1/2 cup coconut oil (melted)
- 1/2 cup almond butter
- 1/4 cup cocoa powder
- 2 tbsp low-calorie sweetener (such as stevia or erythritol)
- 1 tsp vanilla extract
- Pinch of salt

STEP-BY-STEP INSTRUCTIONS:
1. Combine melted coconut oil, almond butter, cocoa powder, sweetener, vanilla extract, and salt in a mixing dish.
2. Spoon the mixture into silicone molds or form into bite-sized balls.
3. Place in the freezer for 10-15 minutes or until stiff.
4. Keep fat bombs in an airtight container in the fridge or freezer until ready to eat.

BENEFITS:

Fat bombs offer rapid energy and are a practical method to boost healthy fat intake on a ketogenic diet.

NUTRITION PLAN: PER SERVING
Calories: 100, Protein: 2g, Fat: 10g, Carbohydrates: 2g

KETO STUFFED MINI BELL PEPPERS

COOKING TIME: 25 MINUTES, SERVING: 4 SERVINGS

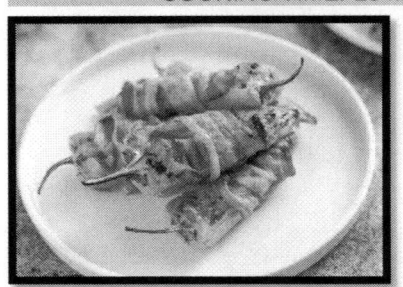

A colorful and filling snack can be made by halving little bell peppers and stuffing them with cream cheese, shredded cheddar cheese, and chopped green onions.

INGREDIENTS:
- 12 mini bell peppers
- 4 oz cream cheese (softened)
- 1/2 cup shredded cheddar cheese
- Two green onions (chopped)
- Salt and pepper to taste

STEP-BY-STEP INSTRUCTIONS:
1. Turn the oven on to 375°F, or 190°C.
2. Remove the seeds after slicing tiny bell peppers in half lengthwise.
3. Combine cream cheese, cheddar cheese, green onions, salt, and pepper in a bowl.
4. Pour the cheese mixture into each half of the pepper.
5. After placing the filled peppers on a baking sheet, bake them for 15 to 20 minutes or until the cheese is bubbling and melted.
6. Warm up and serve.

BENEFITS:
This snack is nutrient-dense and filling because bell peppers are high in antioxidants and vitamin C, while cheese adds calcium and protein.

NUTRITION PLAN: PER SERVING
Calories: 150, Protein: 5g, Fat: 10g, Carbohydrates: 5g

KETO ZUCCHINI CHIPS

COOKING TIME: 30 MINUTES, SERVING: 4 SERVINGS

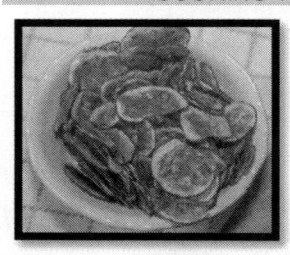

A low-carb, crunchy snack can be made using thinly sliced zucchini rounds seasoned with salt and pepper and baked until crispy.

INGREDIENTS:
- Two medium zucchinis
- 2 tbsp olive oil
- Salt and pepper to taste

STEP-BY-STEP INSTRUCTIONS:
1. Turn the oven on to 225°F, or 110°C.
2. Using a mandoline slicer or knife, thinly slice zucchini.
3. Paint the zucchini slices dry using a paper towel to absorb any remaining moisture.
4. Arrange the slices of zucchini on a parchment paper-lined baking sheet.

5. Season with salt and pepper and drizzle with olive oil.
6. Bake the chips for one to two hours or until crisp and browned.
7. Let the chips cool fully before distributing them.

BENEFITS:
These chips are a healthy substitute for regular potato chips because zucchini is high in fiber and minerals and low in calories and carbs.

NUTRITION PLAN: PER SERVING
Calories: 100, Protein: 2g, Fat: 8g, Carbohydrates: 5g

KETO BUFFALO CHICKEN DIP

COOKING TIME: 30 MINUTES, SERVING: 4 SERVINGS

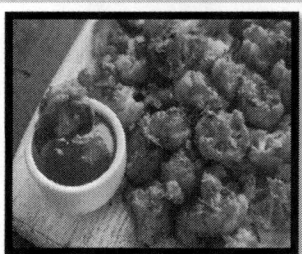

Cream cheese, spicy sauce, ranch dressing, and shredded chicken are combined, baked until bubbling, and then served with celery sticks for dipping.

INGREDIENTS:
- 2 cups shredded chicken
- 8 oz cream cheese (softened)
- 1/2 cup hot sauce
- 1/4 cup ranch dressing
- Celery sticks for serving

STEP-BY-STEP INSTRUCTIONS:
1. Set oven temperature to 175°C/350°F.
2. Shredded chicken, cream cheese, spicy sauce, and ranch dressing should all be thoroughly mixed in a mixing bowl.
3. Spread the mixture evenly in the baking dish after transferring.
4. Bake the dip for 20 to 25 minutes or until it's bubbling and heated.
5. Accompany with celery sticks for dunks.

BENEFITS:
This dip's chicken and cream cheese offer decent protein, and the spicy sauce adds taste without adding unnecessary calories.

NUTRITION PLAN: PER SERVING
Calories: 250, Protein: 15g, Fat: 20g, Carbohydrates: 4g

KETO PECAN PIE BARS

COOKING TIME: 1 HOUR 30 MINUTES, SERVING: 8 SERVINGS

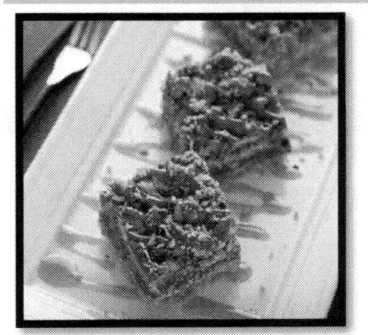

A sweet and crunchy keto dessert made with roasted nuts, butter, and a low-calorie sweetener, spread on parchment paper, then refrigerated until stiff before breaking into pieces.

INGREDIENTS:
- 1 cup pecans
- 1/4 cup butter
- 2 tbsp low-calorie sweetener (such as stevia or erythritol)
- 1/2 tsp vanilla extract
- Pinch of salt

STEP-BY-STEP INSTRUCTIONS:
1. Preheat the oven to 325°F (160° C).
2. Spread the pecans on a baking sheet and toast in the oven for 8-10 minutes until aromatic.
3. Melt the butter in a saucepan over medium heat. Mix in the sweetener, vanilla extract, and salt until smooth.
4. Stir in the toasted pecans until uniformly coated with butter.
5. Line a baking sheet with parchment paper and spread the pecan mixture evenly.
6. Refrigerate for one hour or until stiff.
7. Once hard, crumble the pecan bark into pieces and serve.

BENEFITS:
Pecans are high in healthy fats and antioxidants, and the low-calorie sweetener provides a sweet taste without additional sweets.

NUTRITION PLAN: PER SERVING
Calories: 200, Protein: 2g, Fat: 20g, Carbohydrates: 3g

KETO SOUP RECIPES

KETO CHICKEN ZOODLE SOUP

COOKING TIME: 30 MINUTES, SERVING: 6 SERVINGS

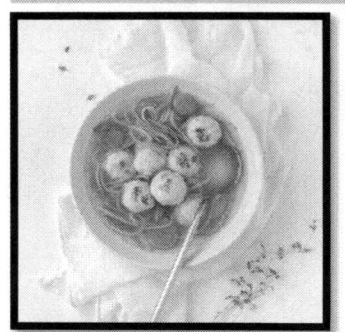

This hearty soup is cooked in a tasty chicken broth with shredded chicken, zucchini noodles, carrots, celery, and onions.

INGREDIENTS:
- 1 lb chicken breasts, cooked and shredded
- Two medium zucchinis noodles sliced
- Two carrots diced
- Two stalks of celery, diced
- One onion, diced
- 6 cups chicken broth
- Salt and pepper to taste
- Optional: chopped fresh parsley for garnish

STEP-BY-STEP INSTRUCTIONS:
1. Saute the onion, celery, and carrots in a big pot until tender.
2. To the pot, add the chicken broth and shreds.
3. Simmer for ten minutes after bringing to a simmer.
4. Add the zucchini and simmer for five minutes when the noodles are cooked.
5. To taste, add salt and pepper for seasoning.
6. If desired, top the hot dish with chopped parsley.

BENEFITS:
This soup is an excellent fit for Dr. Nowzaradan's diet plan since it is low in calories and carbs and high in protein from chicken and veggies, which provide essential nutrients.

NUTRITION PLAN: PER SERVING
Calories: 150, Protein: 20g, Fat: 4g, Carbohydrates: 8g

KETO CREAM OF BROCCOLI SOUP

COOKING TIME: 40 MINUTES, SERVING: 4 SERVINGS

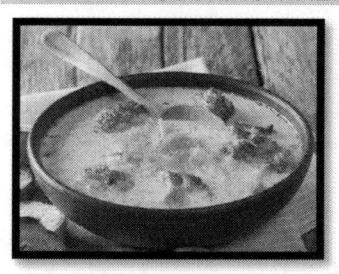

A delicious and filling low-carb soup made with pureed broccoli, heavy cream, and sharp cheddar cheese.

INGREDIENTS:
- ☐ 4 cups broccoli florets
- ☐ 2 cups chicken broth
- ☐ 1 cup heavy cream
- ☐ 1 cup shredded sharp cheddar cheese
- ☐ Salt and pepper to taste

STEP-BY-STEP INSTRUCTIONS:
1. Bring the chicken stock to a boil in a big pot.
2. Add the broccoli florets and boil for ten to fifteen minutes or until tender.
3. Puree the broccoli and broth in a conventional or immersion blender until smooth.
4. Put the pureed mixture back into the pot and toss the shredded cheddar cheese and heavy cream until the cheese melts.
5. To taste, add salt and pepper for seasoning.
6. Warm up the food.

BENEFITS:
This soup is a wholesome and satisfying choice for Dr. Nowzaradan's diet plan since broccoli is high in vitamins and minerals and because heavy cream and cheese contribute satiating lipids.

NUTRITION PLAN: PER SERVING
Calories: 250, Protein: 10g, Fat: 20g, Carbohydrates: 8g

KETO BEEF AND CABBAGE SOUP

COOKING TIME: 45 MINUTES, SERVING: 6 SERVINGS

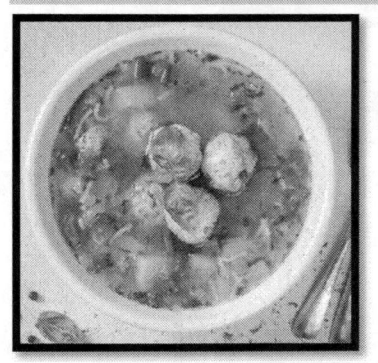

Diced tomatoes, chopped cabbage, and spices are simmered with ground beef to create a substantial and satisfying keto-friendly soup.

INGREDIENTS:
- ☐ 1 lb ground beef
- ☐ 4 cups chopped cabbage
- ☐ One can of diced tomatoes
- ☐ 6 cups beef broth
- ☐ One onion, diced
- ☐ Two cloves garlic, minced
- ☐ 1 tsp paprika
- ☐ Salt and pepper to taste

STEP-BY-STEP INSTRUCTIONS:
1. Brown the ground beef in a large pot over medium heat.
2. Cook the garlic and onion until they become tender.
3. Add the diced tomatoes, paprika, beef broth, chopped cabbage, and salt and pepper to taste.
4. Bring to a simmer and cook until the cabbage is soft for 20 to 25 minutes.
5. Taste and adjust the seasoning.

6. Warm up the food.

BENEFITS:
This soup is a filling and healthy choice for Dr. Nowzaradan's diet plan because it contains protein from the ground beef and nutrients from the cabbage and tomatoes.

NUTRITION PLAN: PER SERVING
Calories: 200, Protein: 15g, Fat: 10g, Carbohydrates: 8g

KETO CAULIFLOWER CHEESE SOUP
COOKING TIME: 35 MINUTES, SERVING: 4 SERVINGS

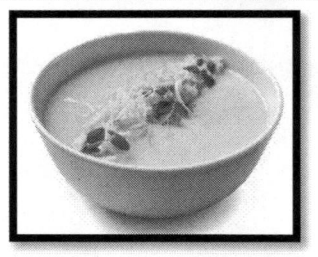

A satisfying low-carb supper of velvety soup made with pureed cauliflower, heavy cream, and sharp cheddar cheese.

INGREDIENTS:
- One medium-head cauliflower, chopped
- 2 cups chicken broth
- 1 cup heavy cream
- 1 cup shredded sharp cheddar cheese
- Salt and pepper to taste

STEP-BY-STEP INSTRUCTIONS:
1. Combine the cauliflower and chicken stock in a large pot.
2. After bringing it to a boil, lower the heat and simmer the cauliflower for 15 to 20 minutes or until it becomes soft.
3. Puree the cauliflower and broth in a conventional blender or with an immersion blender until creamy.
4. Put the pureed mixture back into the pot and toss the shredded cheddar cheese and heavy cream until the cheese melts.
5. To taste, add salt and pepper for seasoning.
6. Warm up the food.

BENEFITS:
This soup is rich and satiating, and it fits in perfectly with Dr. Nowzaradan's diet plan because cauliflower is low in carbs but high in fiber and nutrients.

NUTRITION PLAN: PER SERVING
Calories: 300, Protein: 10g, Fat: 25g, Carbohydrates: 8g

KETO CHICKEN AND MUSHROOM SOUP
COOKING TIME: 40 MINUTES, SERVING: 4 SERVINGS

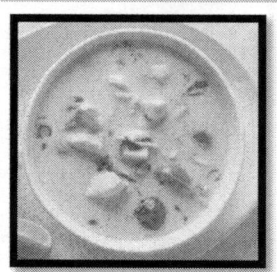

Sliced mushrooms sautéed with garlic and thyme, simmered with shredded chicken and chicken broth

INGREDIENTS:
- 1 lb chicken breasts, cooked and shredded
- 8 oz mushrooms, sliced
- 4 cups chicken broth
- Two cloves garlic, minced
- 1 tsp dried thyme
- Salt and pepper to taste

STEP-BY-STEP INSTRUCTIONS:
1. Sliced mushrooms should be cooked till golden brown in a big pot.
2. When aromatic, add the minced garlic and dry thyme.
3. Add chicken broth and shreds of chicken and stir.
4. Simmer and cook for ten to fifteen minutes.
5. To taste, add salt and pepper for seasoning.
6. Warm up the food.

BENEFITS:
This soup is tasty and nourishing for Dr. Nowzaradan's diet. Mushrooms are low in calories but high in minerals and antioxidants; chicken adds protein.

NUTRITION PLAN: PER SERVING
Calories: 200, Protein: 20g, Fat: 5g, Carbohydrates: 6g

KETO ITALIAN SAUSAGE SOUP
COOKING TIME: 45 MINUTES, SERVING: 6 SERVINGS

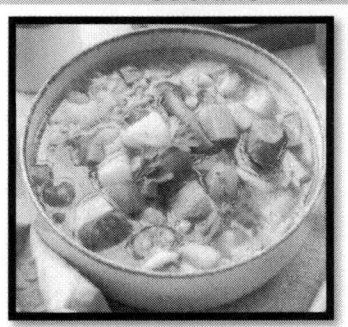

This substantial and filling keto soup is made.

INGREDIENTS:
- 1 lb Italian sausage, casings removed
- One can of diced tomatoes
- 4 cups chicken broth
- 2 cups fresh spinach
- One zucchini, diced
- One onion, diced
- Two cloves garlic, minced
- 1 tsp Italian seasoning
- Salt and pepper to taste

STEP-BY-STEP INSTRUCTIONS:
1. Italian sausage should be browned in a big saucepan over medium heat, breaking it up as it cooks.
2. Cook the minced garlic and diced onion until they are tender.
3. Add the diced zucchini, chicken stock, tomatoes (with liquids), and Italian spice.
4. Once the zucchini is soft, boil it for 15 to 20 minutes at a simmer.
5. Cook the fresh spinach until it wilts.
6. To taste, add salt and pepper for seasoning.
7. Warm up the food.

BENEFITS:
This soup is a substantial and filling choice for Dr. Nowzaradan's diet plan since it contains protein from Italian sausage and nutrients from veggies like spinach and zucchini.

NUTRITION PLAN: PER SERVING
Calories: 250, Protein: 15g, Fat: 15g, Carbohydrates: 8g

KETO CREAMY ASPARAGUS SOUP

COOKING TIME: 30 MINUTES, SERVING: 4 SERVINGS

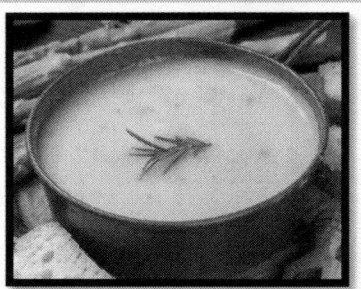

Tender asparagus blended with heavy cream, Parmesan cheese, and garlic for a smooth and creamy low-carb soup.

INGREDIENTS:
- 1 lb asparagus, trimmed and chopped
- 2 cups chicken broth
- 1 cup heavy cream
- 1/4 cup grated Parmesan cheese
- Two cloves garlic, minced
- Salt and pepper to taste

STEP-BY-STEP INSTRUCTIONS:
1. Bring the chicken stock to a boil in a big pot.
2. Add the chopped asparagus and minced garlic, and simmer for 10 to 15 minutes or until the asparagus is soft.
3. Puree the asparagus and broth in a conventional blender or with an immersion blender until smooth.
4. Put the pureed mixture back into the pot and stir in the grated Parmesan cheese and heavy cream until the cheese melts.
5. To taste, add salt and pepper for seasoning.
6. Warm up the food.

BENEFITS:
While heavy cream and Parmesan cheese give this creamy soup richness and flavor, asparagus is low in calories but high in fiber, vitamins, and antioxidants, making it a wholesome option for Dr. Nowzaradan's diet plan.

NUTRITION PLAN: PER SERVING
Calories: 200, Protein: 5g, Fat: 15g, Carbohydrates: 6g

KETO SEAFOOD CHOWDER

COOKING TIME: 45 MINUTES, SERVING: 4 SERVINGS

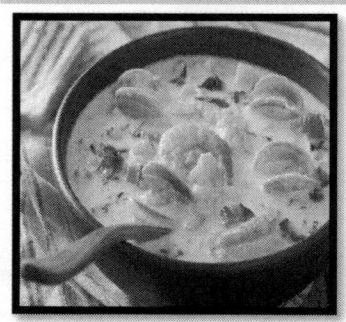

A delectable and low-carb seafood soup, this rich and creamy chowder.

INGREDIENTS:
- 1/2 lb shrimp, peeled and deveined
- 1/2 lb scallops
- 1/2 lb firm white fish, diced
- 4 cups chicken broth
- 1 cup heavy cream
- 4 tbsp butter
- 1/4 cup lemon juice
- Salt and pepper to taste

STEP-BY-STEP INSTRUCTIONS:
1. Melt butter in a big pot over a medium heat.
2. Add the shrimp, scallops, and chopped fish when the seafood is opaque and fully cooked.
3. Add lemon juice, heavy cream, and chicken broth and stir.

4. Simmer and cook for ten to fifteen minutes.
5. To taste, add salt and pepper for seasoning.
6. Warm up the food.

BENEFITS:
The addition of heavy cream enhances this chowder's creaminess and richness, making it a delicious and gratifying alternative to Dr. Nowzaradan's diet plan. Seafood is high in protein, omega-3 fatty acids, and other essential nutrients.

NUTRITION PLAN: PER SERVING
Calories: 300, Protein: 20g, Fat: 20g, Carbohydrates: 5g

MEAL PLAN CHARTS FOR 30 DAYS

Here's a 30-day meal plan incorporating the provided keto breakfast, lunch, dinner, snack, and soup recipes, aligned with Dr. Nowzaradan's dietary guidelines:

S/N	TIME	RECIPES
01	BREAKFAST	Keto Avocado Egg Cups
	LUNCH	Keto Chicken Salad Lettuce Wraps
	DINNER	Keto Baked Salmon with Lemon Butter Sauce
	SNACK	Keto Cheese Crisps
02	BREAKFAST	Spinach and Mushroom Crustless Quiche
	LUNCH	Keto Taco Salad
	DINNER	Keto Garlic Butter Shrimp Scampi
	SNACK	Keto Guacamole with Veggie Sticks
03	BREAKFAST	Zucchini Fritters with Sour Cream
	LUNCH	Keto Egg Roll in a Bowl
	DINNER	Keto Chicken Alfredo Zoodles
	SNACK	Keto Deviled Eggs
04	BREAKFAST	Egg and Bacon Muffin Cups
	LUNCH	Keto Cauliflower Fried Rice
	DINNER	Keto Stuffed Bell Peppers
	SNACK	Keto Fat Bombs
05	BREAKFAST	Cauliflower Breakfast Hash
	LUNCH	Keto Avocado Tuna Salad
	DINNER	Keto Beef and Broccoli Stir-Fry
	SNACK	Keto Zucchini Chips
06	BREAKFAST	Keto Chia Pudding
	LUNCH	Keto Turkey and Cheese Roll-Ups
	DINNER	Keto Eggplant Parmesan
	SNACK	Keto Buffalo Chicken Dip
07	BREAKFAST	Keto Green Smoothie
	LUNCH	Keto Greek Salad with Grilled Chicken
	DINNER	Keto Spaghetti Squash with Meatballs
	SNACK	Keto Pecan Pie Bark
08	BREAKFAST	Keto Avocado Egg Cups
	LUNCH	Keto Chicken Salad Lettuce Wraps
	DINNER	Keto Cauliflower Crust Pizza
	SNACK	Keto Cheese Crisps
09	BREAKFAST	Spinach and Mushroom Crustless Quiche
	LUNCH	Keto Egg Roll in a Bowl
	DINNER	Keto Chicken Alfredo Zoodles
	SNACK	Keto Guacamole with Veggie Sticks

Day	Meal	Dish
10	BREAKFAST	Zucchini Fritters with Sour Cream
	LUNCH	Keto Turkey Club Lettuce Wraps
	DINNER	Keto Beef and Broccoli Stir-Fry
	SNACK	Keto Deviled Eggs
11	BREAKFAST	Egg and Bacon Muffin Cups
	LUNCH	Keto Taco Salad
	DINNER	Keto Stuffed Bell Peppers
	SNACK	Keto Fat Bombs
12	BREAKFAST	Cauliflower Breakfast Hash
	LUNCH	Keto Avocado Tuna Salad
	DINNER	Keto Garlic Butter Shrimp Scampi
	SNACK	Keto Zucchini Chips
13	BREAKFAST	Keto Chia Pudding
	LUNCH	Keto Chicken Salad Lettuce Wraps
	DINNER	Keto Eggplant Parmesan
	SNACK	Keto Buffalo Chicken Dip
14	BREAKFAST	Keto Green Smoothie
	LUNCH	Keto Greek Salad with Grilled Chicken
	DINNER	Keto Spaghetti Squash with Meatballs
	SNACK	Keto Pecan Pie Bark
15	BREAKFAST	Keto Avocado Egg Cups
	LUNCH	Keto Chicken Salad Lettuce Wraps
	DINNER	Keto Cauliflower Crust Pizza
	SNACK	Keto Cheese Crisps
16	BREAKFAST	Spinach and Mushroom Crustless Quiche
	LUNCH	Keto Egg Roll in a Bowl
	DINNER	Keto Chicken Alfredo Zoodles
	SNACK	Keto Guacamole with Veggie Sticks
17	BREAKFAST	Zucchini Fritters with Sour Cream
	LUNCH	Keto Turkey Club Lettuce Wraps
	DINNER	Keto Beef and Broccoli Stir-Fry
	SNACK	Keto Deviled Eggs
18	BREAKFAST	Egg and Bacon Muffin Cups
	LUNCH	Keto Taco Salad
	DINNER	Keto Stuffed Bell Peppers
	SNACK	Keto Fat Bombs
19	BREAKFAST	Cauliflower Breakfast Hash
	LUNCH	Keto Avocado Tuna Salad
	DINNER	Keto Garlic Butter Shrimp Scampi
	SNACK	Keto Zucchini Chips
20	BREAKFAST	Keto Chia Pudding
	LUNCH	Keto Chicken Salad Lettuce Wraps
	DINNER	Keto Eggplant Parmesan
	SNACK	Keto Buffalo Chicken Dip
21	BREAKFAST	Keto Green Smoothie
	LUNCH	Keto Greek Salad with Grilled Chicken
	DINNER	Keto Spaghetti Squash with Meatballs
	SNACK	Keto Pecan Pie Bark
22	BREAKFAST	Keto Avocado Egg Cups
	LUNCH	Keto Chicken Salad Lettuce Wraps
	DINNER	Keto Cauliflower Crust Pizza
	SNACK	Keto Cheese Crisps

Day	Meal	Dish
23	BREAKFAST	Spinach and Mushroom Crustless Quiche
23	LUNCH	Keto Egg Roll in a Bowl
23	DINNER	Keto Chicken Alfredo Zoodles
23	SNACK	Keto Guacamole with Veggie Sticks
24	BREAKFAST	Zucchini Fritters with Sour Cream
24	LUNCH	Keto Turkey Club Lettuce Wraps
24	DINNER	Keto Beef and Broccoli Stir-Fry
24	SNACK	Keto Deviled Eggs
25	BREAKFAST	Egg and Bacon Muffin Cups
25	LUNCH	Keto Taco Salad
25	DINNER	Keto Stuffed Bell Peppers
25	SNACK	Keto Fat Bombs
26	BREAKFAST	Cauliflower Breakfast Hash
26	LUNCH	Keto Avocado Tuna Salad
26	DINNER	Keto Garlic Butter Shrimp Scampi
26	SNACK	Keto Zucchini Chips
27	BREAKFAST	Keto Chia Pudding
27	LUNCH	Keto Chicken Salad Lettuce Wraps
27	DINNER	Keto Eggplant Parmesan
27	SNACK	Keto Buffalo Chicken Dip
28	BREAKFAST	Keto Green Smoothie
28	LUNCH	Keto Greek Salad with Grilled Chicken
28	DINNER	Keto Spaghetti Squash with Meatballs
28	SNACK	Keto Pecan Pie Bark
29	BREAKFAST	Keto Avocado Egg Cups
29	LUNCH	Keto Chicken Salad Lettuce Wraps
29	DINNER	Keto Cauliflower Crust Pizza
29	SNACK	Keto Cheese Crisps
30	BREAKFAST	Spinach and Mushroom Crustless Quiche
30	LUNCH	Keto Egg Roll in a Bowl
30	DINNER	Keto Chicken Alfredo Zoodles
30	SNACK	Keto Guacamole with Veggie Sticks

RECIPES SUITABLE FOR DR. NOWZARADAN'S DIET

Here are eight recipes for each meal category, all suitable for Dr. Nowzaradan's diet, emphasizing low-calorie, high-protein, and nutrient-dense foods.

BREAKFAST RECIPES:

VEGGIE EGG WHITE SCRAMBLE

COOKING TIME: 15 MINUTES, SERVING: 2 SERVINGS

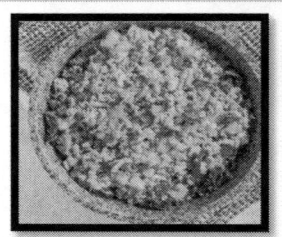

Scrambled egg whites combined with chopped onions, bell peppers, spinach, and a small feta cheese.

INGREDIENTS:
- Eight egg whites,
- 1/2 cup diced bell peppers,
- 1/4 cup diced onions,
- 1 cup chopped spinach,
- Two tablespoons crumbled feta cheese.

STEP-BY-STEP INSTRUCTIONS:
1. A nonstick skillet should be heated to medium heat.
2. Simmer the chopped onions and bell peppers in the skillet until they are tender.
3. When the spinach begins to wilt, add it.
4. Add the egg whites and scramble until thoroughly done.
5. Top with feta cheese and serve warm.

BENEFITS:
Rich in protein and minerals from vegetables, low in calories and carbs.

NUTRITION PLAN: PER SERVING
Calories: 120, Protein: 18g, Fat: 2g, Carbohydrates: 6g

BERRY SMOOTHIE BOWL

COOKING TIME: 5 MINUTES, SERVING: 1 SERVING

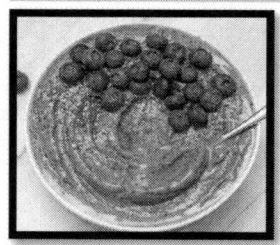

Greek yogurt, spinach, mixed berries, and chia seeds are combined to make a smoothie bowl.

INGREDIENTS:
- 1 cup Greek yogurt,
- 1/2 cup mixed berries,
- 1/2 cup spinach,
- One tablespoon of chia seeds.

STEP-BY-STEP INSTRUCTIONS:
1. Blend spinach, mixed berries, and Greek yogurt in a blender. Process till smooth.
2. Transfer the blended drink to a bowl.
3. If preferred, top with extra berries and a sprinkling of chia seeds.

BENEFITS:
Low in calories and carbs, high in antioxidants, fiber, and protein.

NUTRITION PLAN: PER SERVING
Calories: 180, Protein: 20g, Fat: 3g, Carbohydrates: 18g

SPINACH AND TOMATO FRITTATA
COOKING TIME: 30 MINUTES, SERVING: 4 SERVINGS

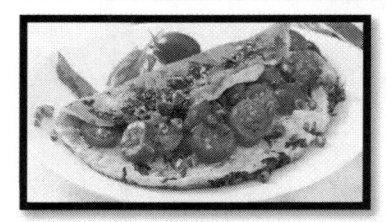

A cooked frittata topped with cherry tomatoes, fresh spinach, and Parmesan cheese.

INGREDIENTS:
- Six eggs
- 1 cup fresh spinach,
- 1/2 cup cherry tomatoes (halved),
- 1/4 cup grated Parmesan cheese.

STEP-BY-STEP INSTRUCTIONS:
1. Set the oven's temperature to 175°C/350°F.
2. Whisk the eggs and Parmesan cheese in a mixing basin.
3. In an oven-safe skillet, preheat the heat to medium. Cook the spinach until it wilts then add the cherry tomatoes.
4. Cover the spinach and tomatoes with the egg mixture. Cook until the edges start to set, a few minutes.
5. After transferring the skillet to the oven, warm it and bake for ten to fifteen minutes or until the frittata is set through.
6. Cut into pieces and present warm.

BENEFITS:
Low in carbohydrates, high in protein, and bursting with vitamins from tomatoes and spinach.

NUTRITION PLAN: PER SERVING
Calories: 130, Protein: 10g, Fat: 8g, Carbohydrates: 4g

GREEK YOGURT WITH NUTS AND SEEDS
COOKING TIME: 5 MINUTES, SERVING: 1 SERVING

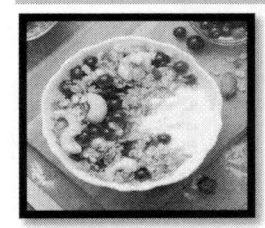

Almonds, sunflower seeds, and flaxseeds combined with plain Greek yogurt to give crunch and protein.

INGREDIENTS:
- 1 cup plain Greek yogurt,
- One tablespoon of almonds,
- One tablespoon of sunflower seeds,
- One teaspoon of flaxseeds.

STEP-BY-STEP INSTRUCTIONS:
1. Fill a bowl with Greek yogurt.
2. Sprinkle almonds, flaxseeds, and sunflower seeds on top.
3. Savor without alteration or top with honey if preferred.

BENEFITS:

It is packed with protein and good fats, adding crunch and minerals to a balanced meal.

NUTRITION PLAN: PER SERVING

Per servingCalories: 220, Protein: 20g, Fat: 10g, Carbohydrates: 10g

OVERNIGHT CHIA PUDDING

PREP: 5 MINUTES, OVERNIGHT SOAK, SERVING: 2 SERVINGS

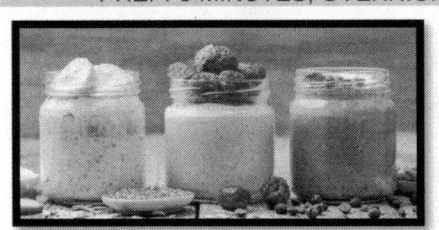

Overnight soaked chia seeds in almond milk, topped with fresh berries and slightly sweetened with vanilla flavor.

INGREDIENTS:
- 1/4 cup chia seeds,
- 1 cup almond milk,
- 1/2 teaspoon vanilla extract,
- 1/2 cup fresh berries.

STEP-BY-STEP INSTRUCTIONS:
1. Mix the chia seeds, almond milk, and vanilla essence in a basin or container. Mix thoroughly.
2. Refrigerate overnight with a cover on.
3. Before serving in the morning, sprinkle some fresh berries on top.

BENEFITS:

Low in calories and carbs, high in protein, fiber, and omega-3 fatty acids.

NUTRITION PLAN: PER SERVING

Calories: 150, Protein: 6g, Fat: 8g, Carbohydrates: 12g

BAKED APPLE OATMEAL

COOKING TIME: 40 MINUTES, SERVING: 4 SERVINGS

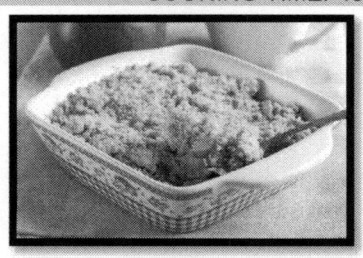

A low-calorie oatmeal that's baked with honey, cinnamon, and diced apples.

INGREDIENTS:
- 2 cups oats,
- Two apples (diced),
- One teaspoon cinnamon,
- Two tablespoons honey,
- 2 cups water.

STEP-BY-STEP INSTRUCTIONS:
1. Turn the oven on to 375°F, or 190°C.
2. Combine the oats, chopped apples, cinnamon, and honey in a baking dish and blend thoroughly.
3. Add the water and mix everything.
4. Bake the oats for 25 to 30 minutes or until it's cooked through and golden brown.
5. Warm up the food.

BENEFITS:

It is rich in fiber, offers a gradual release of energy, and is naturally sweetened with honey and apples.

NUTRITION PLAN: PER SERVING

Calories: 200, Protein: 5g, Fat: 3g, Carbohydrates: 40g

MUSHROOM AND KALE BREAKFAST SKILLET

COOKING TIME: 20 MINUTES, SERVING: 2 SERVINGS

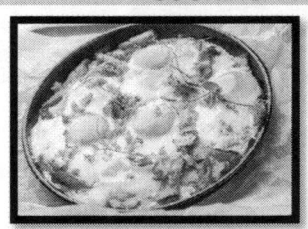

Scrambled eggs, sautéed mushrooms, and greens are combined and finished with a dash of goat cheese.

INGREDIENTS:
- 1 cup sliced mushrooms,
- 1 cup chopped kale,
- Four eggs,
- Two tablespoons of goat cheese.

STEP-BY-STEP INSTRUCTIONS:
1. In a skillet, preheat to medium. Once added, sauté the mushrooms until browned.
2. Cook the kale in the skillet until it wilts.
3. Cover the greens and mushrooms with scrambled eggs. Cook the eggs until they are set.
4. Top with goat cheese and serve warm.

BENEFITS:
Rich in vitamins and minerals from kale and mushrooms, low in calories and carbs, and high in protein and fiber.

NUTRITION PLAN: PER SERVING
Calories: 160, Protein: 14g, Fat: 10g, Carbohydrates: 5g

LUNCH RECIPES

GRILLED CHICKEN AND VEGGIE WRAP

COOKING TIME: 20 MINUTES, SERVING: 2 WRAPS

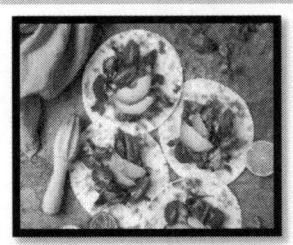

A light tzatziki sauce, cucumbers, mixed greens, and grilled chicken breast are stuffed into a whole-grain wrap.

INGREDIENTS:
- Two whole-grain wraps,
- 1 grilled chicken breast (sliced),
- 1 cup mixed greens,
- 1/2 cucumber (sliced),
- tzatziki sauce (to taste).

STEP-BY-STEP INSTRUCTIONS:
1. Arrange the whole grain wrappers and evenly distribute the sliced cucumber, mixed greens, and grilled chicken breast.
2. Drizzle the fillings with tzatziki sauce.
3. Tightly roll the wraps, cut in half, and proceed to serve.

BENEFITS:
Low in fat and carbs, high in vitamins, fiber, and protein from veggies and chicken.

NUTRITION PLAN: PER SERVING
Calories: 300 (per wrap), Protein: 25g, Fat: 8g, Carbohydrates: 30g

QUINOA AND BLACK BEAN SALAD

COOKING TIME: 20 MINUTES, SERVING: 4 SERVINGS

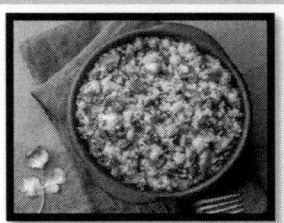

Black beans, corn, sliced bell peppers, and cooked quinoa combined with a lime-cilantro vinaigrette.

INGREDIENTS:
- 1 cup cooked quinoa,
- 1 cup black beans (drained and rinsed),
- 1 cup corn kernels,
- 1/2 cup diced bell peppers,
- lime-cilantro dressing (to taste).

STEP-BY-STEP INSTRUCTIONS:
1. Add the cooked quinoa, black beans, corn, and diced bell peppers to a big bowl.
2. Over the salad, drizzle with the lime-cilantro dressing and toss to mix.
3. Serve at either room temperature or cold.

BENEFITS:
Low in fat and calories, high in fiber and protein from quinoa and black beans, rich in vitamins and minerals from vegetables.

NUTRITION PLAN: PER SERVING
Calories: 250, Protein: 10g, Fat: 3g, Carbohydrates: 45g

CHICKPEA AND CUCUMBER SALAD

COOKING TIME: 15 MINUTES, SERVING: 4 SERVINGS

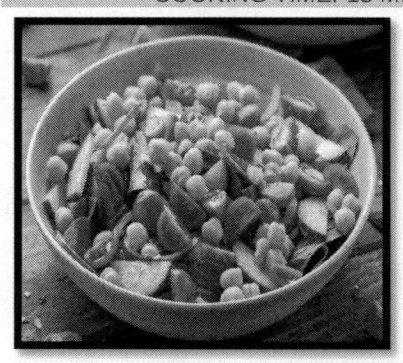

Diced cucumbers, red onion, parsley, and chickpeas combined with lemon juice and olive oil dressing.

INGREDIENTS:
- One can chickpeas (drained and rinsed),
- One cucumber (diced),
- 1/2 red onion (finely chopped),
- 1/4 cup chopped fresh parsley,
- 2 tbsp olive oil,
- Juice of 1 lemon,
- Salt and pepper (to taste).

STEP-BY-STEP INSTRUCTIONS:
1. Combine chickpeas, diced cucumber, chopped red onion, and parsley
2. in a large bowl.
3. Whisk together olive oil, lemon juice, salt, and pepper in a small bowl.
4. Pour the dressing over the chickpea mixture and toss to coat.
5. Serve chilled or at room temperature.

BENEFITS:
High fiber and plant-based protein from chickpeas, rich in vitamins and antioxidants from vegetables, and healthy fats from olive oil.

NUTRITION PLAN: PER SERVING

Calories: 200, Protein: 8g, Fat: 10g, Carbohydrates: 22g

ASIAN CHICKEN LETTUCE WRAPS
COOKING TIME: 20 MINUTES, SERVING: 4 SERVINGS

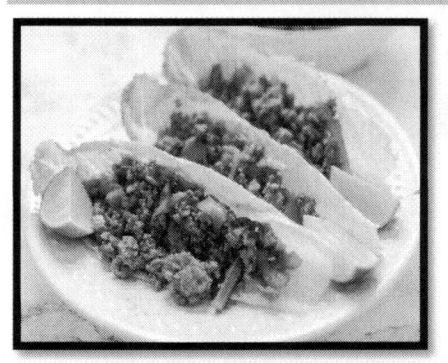

Serve ground chicken sautéed in soy sauce, garlic, and ginger on top of crisp lettuce leaves.

INGREDIENTS:
- 1 lb ground chicken,
- Two cloves garlic (minced),
- 1 inch fresh ginger (grated),
- 2 tbsp low-sodium soy sauce,
- 1 tbsp rice vinegar,
- 1 tsp sesame oil,
- One head of lettuce (leaves separated).

STEP-BY-STEP INSTRUCTIONS:
1. Cook the ground chicken in a big skillet over medium heat until it's browned.
2. Sauté the grated ginger and minced garlic for two more minutes.
3. Add the sesame oil, rice vinegar, and soy sauce. Cook for two to three minutes or until the flavors are well blended.
4. Present the chicken mixture between leaves of lettuce.

BENEFITS:
Rich in vitamins and antioxidants from the lettuce, low in calories and carbs, and high in protein.

NUTRITION PLAN: PER SERVING
Calories: 180, Protein: 20g, Fat: 9g, Carbohydrates: 6g

SHRIMP AND AVOCADO SALAD
COOKING TIME: 20 MINUTES, SERVING: 4 SERVINGS

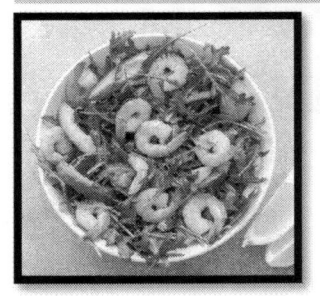

A mild vinaigrette combines cherry tomatoes, avocado, and grilled shrimp.

INGREDIENTS:
- 1 lb shrimp (peeled and deveined),
- Two avocados (diced),
- 2 cups mixed greens,
- 1 cup cherry tomatoes (halved),
- 2 tbsp olive oil,
- 1 tbsp balsamic vinegar,
- Salt and pepper (to taste).

STEP-BY-STEP INSTRUCTIONS:
1. Grill shrimp for 2 to 3 minutes on each side or until they are pink and opaque.
2. Mix mixed greens, chopped avocado, and cherry tomatoes cut in half in a big bowl.
3. Toss the salad with the grilled shrimp.
4. Mix the olive oil, balsamic vinegar, salt, and pepper in a small basin.
5. After drizzling the salad with the vinaigrette, toss to coat.

BENEFITS:
Rich in vitamins and antioxidants from vegetables, low in carbs, high in protein and healthy fats.

NUTRITION PLAN: PER SERVING
Calories: 250, Protein: 20g, Fat: 15g, Carbohydrates: 10g

SPICY LENTIL SOUP

COOKING TIME: 45 MINUTES, SERVING: 4 SERVINGS

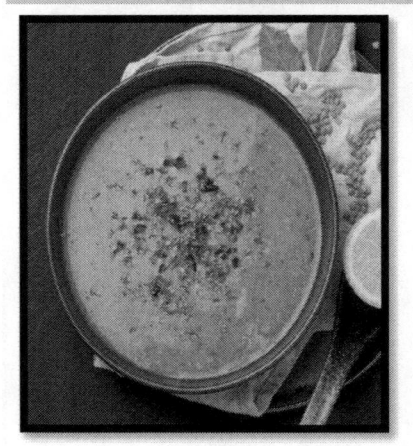

A filling lunch alternative, this soup is composed of lentils, chopped tomatoes, carrots, celery, and a mixture of spices.

INGREDIENTS:
- 1 cup lentils,
- One can of diced tomatoes,
- Two carrots (diced),
- Two celery stalks (diced),
- One onion (diced),
- Two cloves garlic (minced),
- 4 cups vegetable broth,
- 1 tsp cumin,
- 1 tsp paprika,
- 1/2 tsp cayenne pepper,
- salt and pepper (to taste).

STEP-BY-STEP INSTRUCTIONS:
1. Diced carrots, celery, and onion should be sautéed till tender in a big pot.
2. Add the cayenne pepper, cumin, paprika, and minced garlic. Cook for a further two minutes.
3. Add the diced tomatoes, vegetable broth, and lentils and stir.
4. After bringing to a boil, lower the heat and simmer the lentils for 30 to 35 minutes or until soft.
5. To taste, add salt and pepper for seasoning.

BENEFITS:
Rich in veggie vitamins and minerals, low in fat and calories, and high in plant-based protein and fiber.

NUTRITION PLAN: PER SERVING
Calories: 200, Protein: 12g, Fat: 3g, Carbohydrates: 30g

DINNER RECIPES

BAKED COD WITH ROASTED VEGETABLES

TIME: 30-40 MINUTES, SERVING: 4 SERVINGS

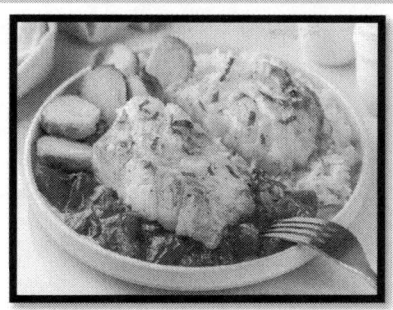

Cod fillets seasoned with lemon and herbs, baked alongside a medley of roasted vegetables.

INGREDIENTS:

- ☐ Four cod fillets, assorted vegetables (such as bell peppers, zucchini, and cherry tomatoes),
- ☐ lemon,
- ☐ herbs (such as thyme or rosemary),
- ☐ olive oil,
- ☐ salt and pepper.

STEP-BY-STEP INSTRUCTIONS:

1. Set oven temperature to 400°F or 200°C.
2. Cod fillets should be placed on a baking pan covered with parchment paper.
3. Place the mixed veggies in a circle around the baking sheet's cod fillets.
4. Season the cod and veggies with salt, pepper, lemon juice, and herbs after drizzling them with olive oil.
5. Bake for 15 to 20 minutes, or until the veggies are soft and the cod is thoroughly cooked, in a preheated oven.

BENEFITS:

Low in calories and carbs, high in protein from the cod, and rich in vitamins and minerals from the veggies.

NUTRITION PLAN: PER SERVING

Calories: 250, Protein: 30g, Fat: 10g, Carbohydrates: 10g

TURKEY AND ZUCCHINI MEATBALLS

COOKING TIME: 30 MINUTES, SERVING: 4 SERVINGS

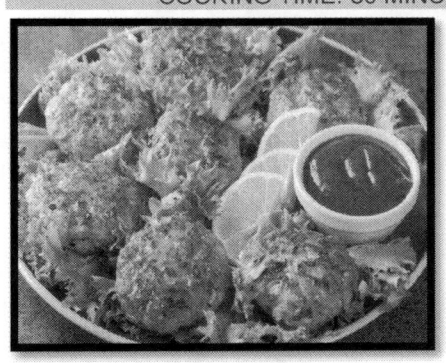

Grated zucchini is combined with lean turkey meatballs, baked, and served with steamed broccoli.

INGREDIENTS:

- ☐ 1 lb ground turkey
- ☐ Two zucchinis (grated)
- ☐ breadcrumbs
- ☐ egg, garlic
- ☐ onion
- ☐ parsley
- ☐ salt, pepper
- ☐ broccoli

STEP-BY-STEP INSTRUCTIONS:

1. Turn the oven on to 375°F, or 190°C.
2. Combine ground turkey, grated zucchini, breadcrumbs, egg, minced garlic, chopped onion, parsley, salt, and pepper in a large bowl.

3. Shape the mixture into meatballs and arrange them on a parchment paper-lined baking sheet.
4. Bake in a warmed oven for 20 to 25 minutes or until the meatballs are thoroughly cooked.
5. Serve the meatballs with a side order of steamed broccoli.

BENEFITS:
Low in calories and carbs, high in protein from the turkey, fiber, and vitamins from the zucchini.

NUTRITION PLAN: PER SERVING
Calories: 200, Protein: 25g, Fat: 8g, Carbohydrates: 8g

STUFFED EGGPLANT BOATS

COOKING TIME: 40-50 MINUTES, SERVING: 4 SERVINGS

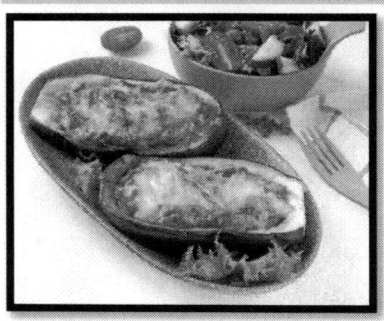

Baked till soft, halved eggplants packed with a mixture of ground chicken, diced tomatoes, and seasonings.

INGREDIENTS:
- Two eggplants
- ground chicken
- diced tomatoes
- onion
- garlic
- spices (such as oregano and basil)
- olive oil.

STEP-BY-STEP INSTRUCTIONS:
1. Turn the oven on to 375°F, or 190°C.
2. Split the eggplants lengthwise in half, then remove the flesh, leaving the shell hollow.
3. Cook ground chicken until thoroughly cooked in a skillet with diced tomatoes, chopped onion, minced garlic, and spices.
4. Spoon the chicken mixture into the hollowed-out eggplant shells.
5. After brushing the stuffed eggplants with olive oil, bake them in the oven for 25 to 30 minutes or until soft.

BENEFITS:
Low in calories and carbs, high in protein from the chicken, fiber, and antioxidants from the tomatoes and eggplant.

NUTRITION PLAN: PER SERVING
Calories: 220, Protein: 20g, Fat: 10g, Carbohydrates: 15g

GARLIC LEMON CHICKEN WITH ASPARAGUS

COOKING TIME: 25-30 MINUTES, SERVING: 4 SERVINGS

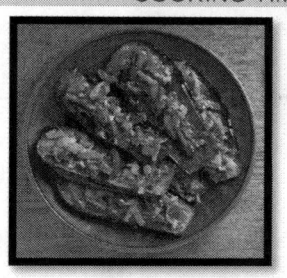

Chicken breast cooked with garlic and lemon served with sautéed asparagus.

INGREDIENTS:
- Four chicken breasts,
- Asparagus spears,
- garlic cloves,
- lemon,
- olive oil,
- salt and pepper.

STEP-BY-STEP INSTRUCTIONS:
1. Add minced garlic, salt, and pepper to chicken breasts for seasoning.
2. In a skillet over medium heat, warm the olive oil. Cook the chicken breasts for 5 to 6 minutes on each side or until they are cooked through and golden brown.
3. Just before the chicken breasts are done, squeeze some fresh lemon juice over them.
4. Sauté asparagus spears in another skillet with olive oil, minced garlic, salt, and pepper until crisp-tender.
5. Garlic lemon chicken should be served with sautéed asparagus on the side.

BENEFITS:
Low in carbs, high in protein from the chicken, and full of vitamins and antioxidants from the asparagus and lemon.

NUTRITION PLAN: PER SERVING
Calories: 250, Protein: 30g, Fat: 10g, Carbohydrates: 8g

SALMON AND SPINACH SALAD

COOKING TIME: 20-25 MINUTES, SERVING: 4 SERVINGS

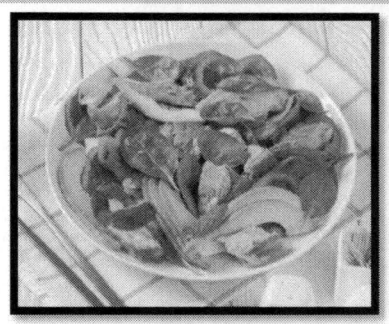

A balsamic vinaigrette, cherry tomatoes, red onion, and spinach accompany a grilled fish fillet.

INGREDIENTS:
- Four salmon fillets,
- Fresh spinach leaves,
- cherry tomatoes,
- red onion,
- balsamic vinegar,
- olive oil,
- salt & pepper.

STEP-BY-STEP INSTRUCTIONS:
1. Rub salmon fillets with olive oil, salt, and pepper. Grill food till it's well done.
2. Combine the thinly sliced red onion, split cherry tomatoes, and fresh spinach leaves in a big bowl.
3. To make the dressing, whisk together olive oil and balsamic vinegar.
4. Top the spinach salad with the grilled salmon fillets and dress with balsamic vinaigrette.

BENEFITS:
Low in carbs, high in protein and omega-3 fatty acids from the salmon, rich in vitamins and minerals from the tomatoes and spinach.

NUTRITION PLAN: PER SERVING
Calories: 300, Protein: 25g, Fat: 15g, Carbohydrates: 10g

BEEF AND VEGETABLE STIR-FRY

COOKING TIME: 20-25 MINUTES, SERVING: 4 SERVINGS

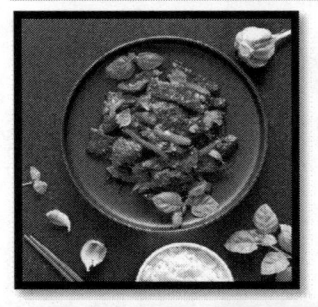

Stir-fried in a light soy sauce with broccoli, bell peppers, and snap peas are lean beef slices.

INGREDIENTS:
- Lean beef strips,
- broccoli florets,
- bell peppers,
- snap peas,
- garlic,
- ginger,
- low-sodium soy sauce.

STEP-BY-STEP INSTRUCTIONS:
1. Over high heat, preheat a wok or large skillet. Stir-fry the beef strips until they turn brown. Take out of the skillet and place aside.
2. Add the chopped garlic, ginger, snap peas, sliced bell peppers, and broccoli florets to the same skillet and stir-fry until the vegetables are crisp-tender.
3. Add low-sodium soy sauce to the skillet with the meat strips once again. Stir-fry until all of the ingredients are well heated.
4. Serve the hot stir-fried beef and vegetables.

BENEFITS:
Low in carbs, high in vitamins and fiber from the veggies, and high in protein from the beef.

NUTRITION PLAN: PER SERVING
Calories: 250, Protein: 30g, Fat: 10g, Carbohydrates: 10g

CAULIFLOWER RICE WITH GRILLED SHRIMP

COOKING TIME: 25-30 MINUTES, SERVING: 4 SERVINGS

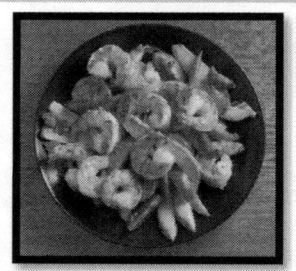

Garlic, herbs, and sautéed cauliflower rice are served with grilled shrimp and lime.

INGREDIENTS:
- Cauliflower,
- shrimp,
- garlic,
- olive oil,
- lime,
- herbs (such as parsley or cilantro).

STEP-BY-STEP INSTRUCTIONS:
1. Grate cauliflower with a grater or food processor until it's rice-sized.

2. In a skillet over medium heat, warm the olive oil. When aromatic, add the minced garlic and sauté it.
3. Cook the cauliflower rice in the skillet for five to seven minutes or until soft.
4. Garlic shrimp till they turn pink and become opaque.
5. Toss the cauliflower rice with herbs, salt, and pepper. Garnish with grilled shrimp and a lime wedge.

BENEFITS:
Rich in protein from the shrimp, fiber, and vitamins from the cauliflower; low in calories and carbs.

NUTRITION PLAN: PER SERVING
Calories: 200, Protein: 25g, Fat: 8g, Carbohydrates: 10g

CHICKEN AND VEGGIE SKEWERS
COOKING TIME: 25-30 MINUTES, SERVING: 4 SERVINGS

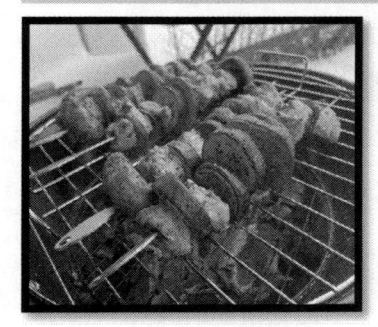

Grilled chicken breast skewers with zucchini, cherry tomatoes, bell peppers, and quinoa sides.

INGREDIENTS:
- ☐ Chicken Breast
- ☐ Zucchini
- ☐ Bell Peppers
- ☐ Cherry Tomatoes
- ☐ Olive Oil
- ☐ Garlic
- ☐ Lemon
- ☐ Quinoa

STEP-BY-STEP INSTRUCTIONS:
1. Cube the chicken breast and thread it onto skewers with cherry tomatoes, bell peppers, and zucchini chunks.
2. After sprinkling the skewers with olive oil, minced garlic, and lemon juice, let them marinate for fifteen to twenty minutes.
3. Grease the grill grates and preheat the grill to medium-high heat.
4. Turn the skewers once or twice while grilling them for 8 to 10 minutes or until the chicken is cooked and the vegetables are soft.
5. As the skewers cook, prepare the quinoa per the directions on the package.
6. Accompany the grilled chicken and vegetable skewers with cooked quinoa on the side.

BENEFITS:
It is low in carbohydrates, fiber and vitamins from the veggies, and protein from the chicken.

NUTRITION PLAN: PER SERVING
Calories: 300, Protein: 25g, Fat: 10g, Carbohydrates: 20g

SNACK RECIPES

MIXED NUTS

TIME: READY TO EAT, SERVING: 1 SERVING (HANDFUL)

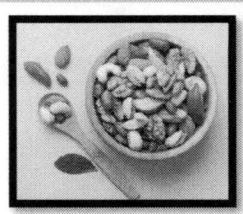

Snacking on a handful of mixed nuts, including cashews, walnuts, and almonds, is a satisfying and healthful snack high in beneficial fats and protein.

INGREDIENTS:
- Almonds,
- walnuts,
- cashews (or any preferred nuts).

STEP-BY-STEP INSTRUCTIONS:
1. Just take a few handfuls of mixed nuts and dig in!

BENEFITS:
Low in carbs, high in vitamins and minerals, and protein and good fats.

NUTRITION PLAN: PER SERVING
Calories: 200, Protein: 7g, Fat: 15g, Carbohydrates: 5g

TUNA SALAD CUCUMBER BITES

COOKING TIME: 15 MINUTES, SERVING: 1 SERVING

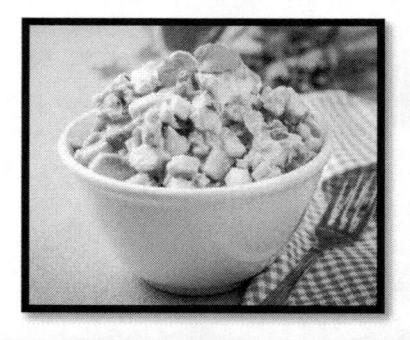

A protein-rich and refreshing snack, cucumber slices can be topped with a dollop of Greek yogurt-based tuna salad with chopped veggies.

INGREDIENTS:
- Cucumber,
- canned tuna,
- Greek yogurt,
- chopped vegetables (such as celery and onion),
- lemon juice,
- salt & pepper.

STEP-BY-STEP INSTRUCTIONS:
1. Cut cucumbers into circles and place them on a platter.
2. To create tuna salad, combine canned tuna, Greek yogurt, finely chopped veggies, lemon juice, salt, and pepper in a bowl.
3. Serve tuna salad by spooning it onto cucumber slices.

BENEFITS:
Low in carbs, high in protein from Greek yogurt and tuna, and pleasant and refreshing.

NUTRITION PLAN: PER SERVING
Calories: 100, Protein: 10g, Fat: 3g, Carbohydrates: 5g

SOUP RECIPES

VEGETABLE SOUP

TIME: 30-45 MINUTES, SERVING: 6 SERVINGS

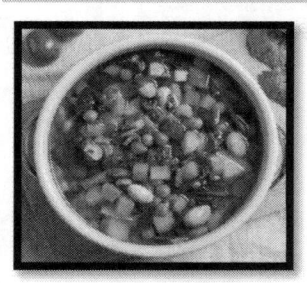

To make a filling, calorie-efficient soup rich in vitamins and minerals yet low in calories, simmer an assortment of vibrant veggies in a tasty broth.

INGREDIENTS:
- Assorted vegetables (such as carrots, celery, onions, bell peppers, and zucchini),
- Vegetable broth,
- Herbs and spices.

STEP-BY-STEP INSTRUCTIONS:
1. Dice the vegetables into small pieces.
2. Add the vegetables to a large pot and sauté until soft.
3. After adding the veggie broth, cook it.
4. Simmer the vegetables for 20 to 30 minutes or until thoroughly cooked.
5. To taste, add more or less herb and spice seasoning.

BENEFITS:
Being high in vitamins and minerals, low in calories, and fiber, and promoting satiety.

NUTRITION PLAN: PER SERVING
Calories: 100, Protein: 3g, Fat: 1g, Carbohydrates: 20g

CHICKEN AND VEGETABLE SOUP

COOKING TIME: 45 MINUTES, SERVING: 6 SERVINGS

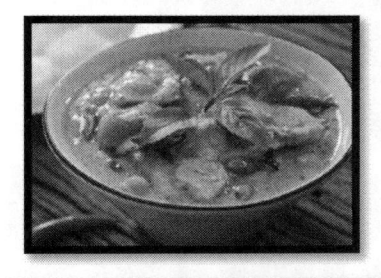

Lean chicken breast, mixed veggies, and herbs make a hearty, high-protein soup ideal for chilly winter days.

INGREDIENTS:
- Chicken breast,
- mixed vegetables (such as carrots, celery, onions, and peas),
- chicken broth,
- herbs and spices.

STEP-BY-STEP INSTRUCTIONS:
1. Cook the chicken breast until it's done, then chop or shred it.
2. Add the vegetables to a large pot and sauté until soft.
3. To the pot, add the chicken broth and shreds.
4. Reduce heat to a simmer and cook for 20 to 30 minutes.
5. To taste, add more or less herb and spice seasoning.

BENEFITS:
Low in calories, high in protein, vitamins, and minerals, and helps with satiety.

NUTRITION PLAN: PER SERVING
Calories: 150, Protein: 15g, Fat: 3g, Carbohydrates: 15g

TOMATO BASIL SOUP
COOKING TIME: 30 MINUTES, SERVING: 4 SERVINGS

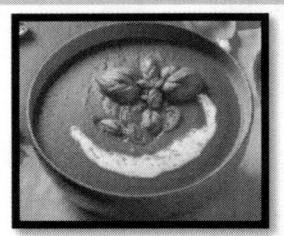

Nutrients that strengthen the immune system and antioxidants.

INGREDIENTS:
- Ripe tomatoes,
- fresh basil,
- garlic,
- vegetable broth,
- olive oil.

STEP-BY-STEP INSTRUCTIONS:
1. Garlic is sautéed in olive oil until aromatic.
2. To the pot, add the chopped tomatoes and vegetable broth.
3. Simmer for around 20 minutes.
4. Puree soup till smooth, then add chopped basil and mix.

BENEFITS:
Rich in immune-boosting minerals, low in calories, and high in antioxidants.

NUTRITION PLAN: PER SERVING
Calories: 80, Protein: 2g, Fat: 3g, Carbohydrates: 10g

MINESTRONE SOUP
COOKING TIME: 60 MINUTES, SERVING: 8 SERVINGS

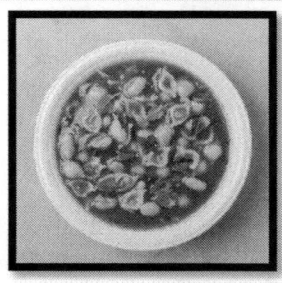

Make a tasty and wholesome dinner with a classic Italian minestrone with veggies, beans, and whole-grain pasta.

INGREDIENTS:
- Mixed vegetables (such as carrots, celery, onions, zucchini, and tomatoes),
- cannellini beans,
- whole-grain pasta,
- vegetable broth,
- herbs and spices.

STEP-BY-STEP INSTRUCTIONS:
1. Celery, carrots, and onions should be sautéed until soft.
2. Add the chopped veggies, pasta, beans, and vegetable broth to the pot.
3. Simmer the pasta and vegetables for 30 to 40 minutes or until thoroughly cooked.
4. To taste, add more or less herb and spice seasoning.

BENEFITS:
Low in calories, high in fiber, vitamins, and minerals, and helps with satiety.

NUTRITION PLAN: PER SERVING
Calories: 150, Protein: 6g, Fat: 1g, Carbohydrates: 30g

SPLIT PEA SOUP

COOKING TIME: 60 MINUTES, SERVING: 6 SERVINGS

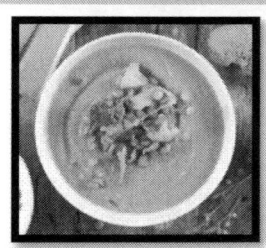

Combine split peas with ham, onions, and carrots to make a hearty, high-protein soup for winter nights.

INGREDIENTS:
- Split peas, onions,
- carrots,
- ham or smoked turkey,
- vegetable broth,
- herbs and spices.

STEP-BY-STEP INSTRUCTIONS:
1. Cook the ham, onions, and carrots until they are soft.
2. Fill the kettle with the vegetable broth and split peas.
3. Simmer until the split peas are tender, and the soup has thickened about 60 to 75 minutes.
4. After the split peas are cooked, add as much or as little herbs and spices to the soup as desired.

BENEFITS:
Low in calories, nutrient-dense, high in protein and fiber from split peas.

NUTRITION PLAN: PER SERVING
Calories: 220, Protein: 15g, Fat: 2g, Carbohydrates: 40g

MUSHROOM BARLEY SOUP

COOKING TIME: 60 MINUTES, SERVING: 6 SERVINGS

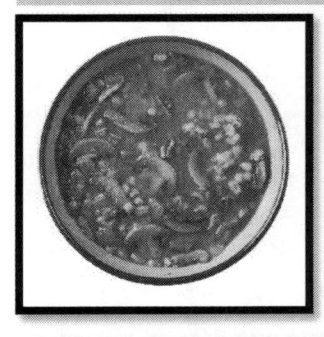

Rich in minerals and fiber, this soup is robust and nourishing, made by simmering earthy mushrooms with barley and aromatic spices.

INGREDIENTS:
- Mushrooms,
- barley,
- onions
- carrots
- celery
- vegetable broth
- herbs and spices

STEP-BY-STEP INSTRUCTIONS:
1. Celery, carrots, and onions should be sautéed until soft.
2. Toss in the barley and chopped mushrooms.
3. After adding the vegetable broth, boil the mixture.
4. Let cook until barley is soft, 45 to 60 minutes.
5. To taste, add more or less herb and spice seasoning.

BENEFITS:
Low in calories, high in minerals and fiber, and encourages satiety.

NUTRITION PLAN: PER SERVING

Calories: 180, Protein: 6g, Fat: 1g, Carbohydrates: 35g

MEAL PLAN CHARTS FOR 30 DAYS

Dr. Nowzaradan's diet typically focuses on low-calorie, high-protein meals. This plan offers around 1200 calories per day.

S/N	TIME	RECIPES
01	BREAKFAST	Veggie Egg White Scramble
	LUNCH	Grilled Chicken and Veggie Wrap
	DINNER	Baked Cod with Roasted Vegetables
	SNACK	Greek Yogurt Parfait
02	BREAKFAST	Berry Smoothie Bowl
	LUNCH	Quinoa and Black Bean Salad
	DINNER	Turkey and Zucchini Meatballs with Steamed Broccoli
	SNACK	Vegetable Sticks with Hummus
03	BREAKFAST	Cottage Cheese with Pineapple
	LUNCH	Tuna and Avocado Salad with Lettuce
	DINNER	Stuffed Eggplant Boats
	SNACK	Hard-Boiled Eggs
04	BREAKFAST	Spinach and Tomato Frittata
	LUNCH	Chickpea and Cucumber Salad
	DINNER	Garlic Lemon Chicken with Asparagus
	SNACK	Cottage Cheese with Pineapple
05	BREAKFAST	Greek Yogurt with Nuts and Seeds
	LUNCH	Asian Chicken Lettuce Wraps
	DINNER	Salmon and Spinach Salad with Balsamic Vinaigrette
	SNACK	Mixed Nuts
06	BREAKFAST	Overnight Chia Pudding
	LUNCH	Spicy Lentil Soup
	DINNER	Beef and Vegetable Stir-Fry with Cauliflower Rice
	SNACK	Turkey and Cheese Roll-Ups
07	BREAKFAST	Baked Apple Oatmeal
	LUNCH	Shrimp and Avocado Salad
	DINNER	Chicken and Veggie Skewers with Quinoa
	SNACK	Tuna Salad Cucumber Bites
08	BREAKFAST	Greek Yogurt with Berries and Chia Seeds
	LUNCH	Chickpea Salad Sandwich on Whole-Wheat Bread
	DINNER	Shrimp Scampi with Zucchini Noodles
	SNACK	Vegetable Sticks with Guacamole
09	BREAKFAST	Scrambled Eggs with Spinach and Mushrooms
	LUNCH	Lentil Soup with a Side Salad
	DINNER	Baked Salmon with Roasted Brussels Sprouts
	SNACK	Cottage Cheese with Sliced Peppers
10	BREAKFAST	Overnight Oats with Almonds and Cinnamon
	LUNCH	Turkey and Veggie Lettuce Wraps
	DINNER	Chicken Stir-Fry with Broccoli and Brown Rice
	SNACK	Greek Yogurt Parfait with Nuts and Honey
11	BREAKFAST	Veggie Egg White Scramble
	LUNCH	Grilled Chicken and Veggie Wrap
	DINNER	Baked Cod with Roasted Vegetables
	SNACK	Greek Yogurt Parfait

Day	Meal	Description
12	BREAKFAST	Smoothie Bowl with Greek Yogurt, Spinach, and Berries
	LUNCH	Tuna Salad with Mixed Greens
	DINNER	Vegetarian Chili with a Dollop of Low-Fat Greek Yogurt
	SNACK	Edamame Pods
13	BREAKFAST	Hard-Boiled Eggs with Avocado Slices
	LUNCH	Quinoa Black Bean Bowl with a Lime Vinaigrette
	DINNER	Turkey Meatloaf with Roasted Vegetables
	SNACK	Carrot Sticks with Hummus
14	BREAKFAST	Baked Apple with a sprinkle of Cinnamon
	LUNCH	Chicken Caesar Salad
	DINNER	Salmon with Lemon and Dill, served with Cauliflower Rice
	SNACK	Greek Yogurt with Berries
15	BREAKFAST	Cottage Cheese Pancakes with Berries (use a low-carb pancake recipe)
	LUNCH	Tofu Scramble with Bell Peppers and Onions (a vegetarian protein option)
	DINNER	Baked Chicken Breast with Roasted Sweet Potato and Green Beans
	SNACK	Celery Sticks with Almond Butter
16	BREAKFAST	Chia Seed Pudding with a splash of Unsweetened Almond Milk and Sliced Almonds
	LUNCH	Turkey and Vegetable Soup
	DINNER	Shrimp Fajitas with Lettuce Wraps (use low-carb tortillas or skip them)
	SNACK	Mixed Nuts and Dried Cranberries (small portion)
17	BREAKFAST	Greek Yogurt with a sprinkle of Granola and Berries
	LUNCH	Chicken Breast Salad with a light vinaigrette dressing
	DINNER	Vegetarian Black Bean Burgers on Whole-Wheat Buns with a side salad
	SNACK	Sliced Cucumber with Cottage Cheese
18	BREAKFAST	Repeat a favorite meal from Week 1 or 2!
	LUNCH	Scrambled Eggs with Smoked Salmon and Spinach
	DINNER	Lentil Salad with chopped vegetables and a lemon-olive oil dressing
	SNACK	Baked Tilapia with Asparagus and Lemon
19	BREAKFAST	Cottage Cheese with Pineapple Chunks
	LUNCH	Oatmeal with Protein Powder and Berries
	DINNER	Tuna Salad Stuffed Avocado
	SNACK	Chicken and Vegetable Stir-Fry with Brown Rice
20	BREAKFAST	Greek Yogurt Parfait with a sprinkle of granola and berries
	LUNCH	Smoothie Bowl with Spinach, Banana, and Protein Powder
	DINNER	Chicken and Black Bean Salad with a side of whole-wheat crackers
	SNACK	Vegetarian Stuffed Peppers with Quinoa and Vegetables
21	BREAKFAST	Edamame Pods with a sprinkle of Sea Salt
	LUNCH	Protein Pancakes with sugar-free syrup (use a low-carb pancake recipe)
	DINNER	Grilled Chicken Caesar Salad with a light dressing
	SNACK	Baked Salmon with Roasted Brussels Sprouts and Quinoa
22	BREAKFAST	Carrot Sticks with Guacamole
	LUNCH	Scrambled Eggs with Tomatoes and Onions
	DINNER	Black Bean Soup with a side salad
	SNACK	Turkey Chili with a dollop of low-fat Greek Yogurt

Day	Meal	Description
23	BREAKFAST	Apple Slices with Almond Butter
	LUNCH	Overnight Oats with Chia Seeds and a splash of unsweetened almond milk
	DINNER	Tuna Salad Lettuce Wraps
	SNACK	Shrimp Scampi with Zucchini Noodles
24	BREAKFAST	Greek Yogurt Parfait with a sprinkle of granola and berries
	LUNCH	Baked Apple with a sprinkle of Cinnamon
	DINNER	Chicken Caesar Salad
	SNACK	Salmon with Lemon and Dill, served with Cauliflower Rice
25	BREAKFAST	Greek Yogurt with Berries
	LUNCH	Cottage Cheese with Sliced Bell Peppers and a drizzle of olive oil
	DINNER	Lentil Salad with a lemon-olive oil dressing
	SNACK	Chicken Stir-Fry with Broccoli and Cauliflower Rice
26	BREAKFAST	Edamame Pods with a sprinkle of Sea Salt
	LUNCH	Smoothie Bowl with Spinach, Berries, and Protein Powder
	DINNER	Chicken and Vegetable Kabobs with a side of hummus
	SNACK	Baked Tilapia with Roasted Asparagus and Lemon
27	BREAKFAST	Celery Sticks with Cream Cheese and Sliced Cucumber
	LUNCH	Scrambled Eggs with Smoked Salmon and Avocado
	DINNER	Chickpea Salad Sandwich on Whole-Wheat Bread
	SNACK	Vegetarian Chili with a side salad
28	BREAKFAST	Cottage Cheese with Pineapple Chunks
	LUNCH	Protein Waffles with Berries and sugar-free syrup (use a low-carb waffle recipe)
	DINNER	Leftover Chicken Kabobs from Day 27 with a side salad
	SNACK	Baked Cod with Lemon and Herbs, served with roasted vegetables
29	BREAKFAST	Vegetable Sticks with Guacamole
	LUNCH	Hard-boiled eggs with Sliced Tomatoes and a sprinkle of herbs
	DINNER	Shrimp and Avocado Salad with a light vinaigrette dressing
	SNACK	Turkey Meatloaf with Mashed Cauliflower (use low-carb alternatives for mashed potatoes)
30	BREAKFAST	Greek Yogurt Parfait with a sprinkle of granola and berries
	LUNCH	Baked Apple with a sprinkle of Cinnamon
	DINNER	Chicken Caesar Salad
	SNACK	Salmon with Lemon and Dill, served with Cauliflower Rice

365-DAY TRACKING JOURNAL FOR WEIGHT LOSS

Welcome to your 365-Day Weight Loss Tracking Journal. This journal will help you track your daily food intake, exercise, and progress toward your weight loss objectives. Consistency is essential; this notebook will help you stay accountable, inspired, and on track throughout the year.

HOW TO USE THIS JOURNAL

DAILY ENTRIES:
Keep track of your meals, snacks, and beverages. Note the portion sizes and any nutritional information available. Track your physical activity, including the type, duration, and intensity.

WEEKLY REFLECTION:
At the end of each week, review your progress. Please take note of any obstacles you encountered, how you overcame them, and which solutions worked best.

MONTHLY REVIEW:
Assess your progress every month. Track your weight, measurements, and other progress indicators, including energy levels, mood, and physical changes.
Set realistic and attainable goals at the beginning of each month. These goals may relate to weight, exercise, eating habits, or mental health.

INSPIRATIONAL QUOTATIONS AND RECOMMENDATIONS:
Throughout the notebook, you will find motivational quotations and recommendations to help you stay inspired and encouraged.

DAILY TRACKING

Daily Tracking

Date: _____ Plan Number: _____ Weight: _____

Goals Archived: _____

Breakfast
_____
_____
_____
_____

Lunch
_____
_____
_____
_____

Water

Dinner
_____
_____
_____
_____

Snacks/Soup
_____
_____
_____
_____

Caffeine

Activities/Exercise
_____
_____
_____
_____

Amount   Notes
_____   _____
_____   _____
_____   _____
_____   _____

Steps

What went well today?
_____
_____
_____

What could be improved?
_____
_____
_____

Sleep

How do you feel?
_____
_____
_____

How to make better tomorrow?
_____
_____
_____

Fitness

Reflection/ Issue / Solve
_____
_____
_____

Issue

Your Quote
_____
_____

Calories

WEEKLY REFLECTION

One Weak Tracking

Dates: _____ to _____ Weak no: _____ Weight Change: _____
Goals Achieved: _____

Dates: _____ Weight: _____ to Date: _____ Weight: _____

Challenges Faced	Strategies for Next Week	Water
_____	_____	
_____	_____	
_____	_____	

Weekly Goals	Missed Goals	Caffeine
_____	_____	
_____	_____	
_____	_____	

Most Activities/Exercise | Amount | Notes | Steps

How do you feel about your progress? | What could be improved? | Sleep

What are you proud of this week? | How to make better Weak? | Fitness

Reflection/ Issue / Solve | | Issue

Your Quote | | Calories

MONTHLY REVIEW

Monthly Tracking

Dates: _____ to _____ Weak no: _____ Weight Change: _____
Goals Achieved: _____

Date: _____   Date: _____
Weight: _____ Waist: _____   Weight: _____ Waist: _____
Hips: _____ Chest: _____   Hips: _____ Chest: _____
Arms: _____ Thighs: _____   Arms: _____ Thighs: _____

Challenges Faced	Strategies for Next Month	Water

Monthly Goals	Missed Goals	Caffeine

Most Activities/Exercise	Amount	Notes	Steps

How do you feel about your progress?	What could be improved?	Sleep

What did you learn this month?	How to make better Month?	Fitness

Reflection/ Issue / Solve   Issue

Your Quote   Calories

365-DAY REFLECTION

Yearly Tracking

Dates: _____ to _____ Weak no: _____ Weight Change: _____
Goals Achieved: _____
_____

Date: _____   Date: _____
Weight: _____ Waist: _____   Weight: _____ Waist: _____
Hips: _____ Chest: _____   Hips: _____ Chest: _____
Arms: _____ Thighs: _____   Arms: _____ Thighs: _____

Challenges Faced	Biggest Challenges	Water
_____	_____	
_____	_____	
_____	_____	

Strategies That Worked	Looking Ahead	Caffeine
_____	_____	
_____	_____	
_____	_____	

Most Activities/Exercise   Amount   Notes   Steps
_____   _____   _____
_____   _____   _____
_____   _____   _____

How will you maintain your   What advice would you give   Sleep
progress?   to others?
_____   _____
_____   _____

Journey changed you?   Your goals for the next year?   Fitness
_____   _____
_____   _____

Final Reflection/ Issue / Solve   Issue
_____
_____

Your Quote   Calories
_____
_____

(163)

90 DAYS TRACKING JOURNAL NOTEBOOK

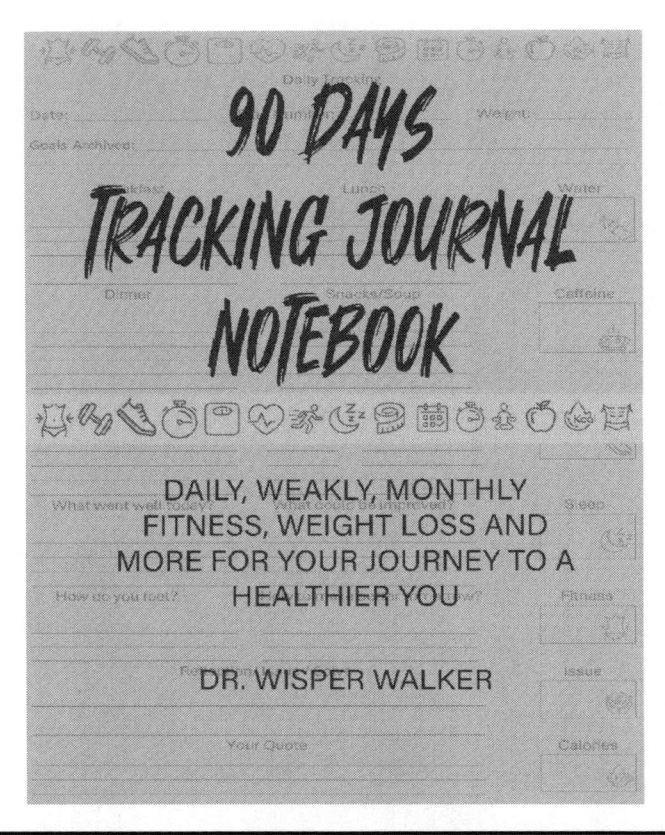

DAILY, WEAKLY, MONTHLY FITNESS, WEIGHT LOSS AND MORE FOR YOUR JOURNEY TO A HEALTHIER YOU

DR. WISPER WALKER

GRAB YOUR 365 DAYS WEIGHTLOSS TRACKING NOTEBOOK

If You want this NoteBook
DIRECT AMAZON LINK

SCAN ME!

HOW TO USE THE 52-WEEK JOURNAL AND THE IMPORTANCE OF TRACKING PROGRESS

Welcome to your 52-week Journal for Tracking Progress! This journal is designed to help you stay organized, motivated, and accountable as you work towards your goals over a year. Tracking your progress is essential for achieving success, and this journal will guide you to stay on track every step of the way.

IMPORTANCE OF TRACKING PROGRESS

Tracking your progress provides several benefits:

Accountability: By recording your daily activities and progress, you hold yourself accountable for your actions.
Motivation: Seeing your progress over time can boost your motivation and inspire you to keep pushing towards your goals.
Identifying Patterns: Tracking allows you to identify patterns in your behavior, both positive and negative, so that you can make necessary adjustments.
Goal Setting: Tracking helps you set realistic and achievable goals based on your progress and results.
Celebrating Success: Reflecting on your progress allows you to celebrate your successes and acknowledge your hard work, no matter how small.

HOW TO USE THE JOURNAL

SETTING GOALS
ESTABLISHING LONG-TERM OBJECTIVES:
You hope to accomplish by the end of the year is an excellent place to start. These objectives must be time-bound, meaningful, quantifiable, achievable, and targeted (SMART).

SHORT-TERM OBJECTIVES:
Divide your long-term objectives into manageable chunks or short-term goals that you may concentrate on every week or month.

EVERY WEEK MONITORING
DAILY LOGS:
Keep track of everything you do every day, such as meals, exercise, water intake, sleep patterns, and any other pertinent data.

WEEKLY OBJECTIVES:
- At the start of each week, establish clear objectives for what you want to accomplish.
- After every week, evaluate your accomplishments, areas for growth, improvement, and any difficulties you encountered.

EVERY MONTH REVIEW
PROGRESS REVIEW:
After every month, evaluate your progress toward your objectives, make any required goal adjustments, and acknowledge your accomplishments.

GOAL-SETTING:
Determine what you want to achieve next and base your following month's goals on your progress.

YEAR-END ANALYSIS
YEAR-END ANALYSIS:
At the end of the year, consider your overall development, accomplishments, and difficulties. Recognize your successes and make plans for the following year.

SUCCESS ADVICE
CONSISTENCY:
To keep focused on your objectives and preserve consistency, develop the daily practice of tracking your progress.
HONESTY:
Be sincere with yourself when documenting your actions and advancement. This will enable you to evaluate your habits correctly and implement significant changes.
POSITIVITY:
Remain upbeat and concentrate on your accomplishments, no matter how minor. Acknowledge your achievements and turn setbacks into teaching moments.
FLEXIBILITY:
Be adaptable and ready to change your plans and objectives. Although you may face unforeseen obstacles, your long-term success depends on your adaptability.

One effective strategy for reaching your objectives and leading a better, happier life is to keep track of your progress. Using this diary, maintain accountability, motivation, and organization on your road toward achievement. Though it could seem sluggish at times, each step you take will get you one step closer to your objectives. Remain dedicated, stay on task, and always keep sight of your goals.